Three 19th-Century Women Doctors

Three 19th-Century Women Doctors

Elizabeth Blackwell
Mary Walker
Sarah Loguen Fraser

written by

Mary K. LeClair
Justin D. White
Susan Keeter, M.F.A.

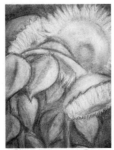

Hofmann Press
Syracuse, New York

On the cover, clockwise from top: Elizabeth Blackwell painted by Joseph Stanley Kozlowski, 1963 (reproduced as U.S. commemorative stamp, 1974.) Collection of SUNY Upstate Medical University, Syracuse, NY; Sarah Loguen Fraser painted by Susan Keeter, 2000. Collection of SUNY Upstate Medical University, Syracuse, NY; Mary Walker painted by Glenora Case Richards (miniature water color on ivory) for the 1982 U.S. commemorative stamp.

Back Cover: Medical student Sarah Loguen assisting in surgery, detail of painting by Susan Keeter.

Elizabeth Blackwell: In the fullest sense of the word a pioneer
© 2007 by Mary K. LeClair. All rights reserved.

Dr. Mary Walker: "A missionary spirit " © 2007 by Justin D. White. All rights reserved.

All the Heaven I Want: The Life of Dr. Sarah Loguen Fraser
© 2007 by Susan Keeter. All rights reserved.

The Hofmann Press gratefully acknowledges the use of material from the following work: *Yankee Women: Gender Battles in the Civil War* by Elizabeth Leonard. Copyright ©1994 by Elizabeth D. Leonard. Used by permission of W. W. Norton & Company, Inc.

Library of Congress Control Number: 2007929350

ISBN: 978-0-9700519-3-6

Contents

Foreword

The three women profiled in this book have at least one thing in common: they persisted. They persisted against huge odds, mostly having to do with gender.

They were in the wrong place at the wrong time.

It's hard, at this distance, imagining how difficult it must have been for Elizabeth Blackwell, Mary Walker and Sarah Loguen Fraser. Considering the talents they possessed, today each would have moved quickly to the top of the medical profession. Just like 19th-century immigrants in a strange land, they applied their unique personalities to the challenge.

And each, in their different ways, won. They left their own, particular marks.

Elizabeth Blackwell was our first woman physician. Mary Walker was involved in politics as well as medicine. Sarah Loguen Fraser was one of the nation's first African American women doctors. Each spent a lifetime going against the grain; at the end of her life, Dr. Fraser may have had an easier time of it than Elizabeth Blackwell, who died being able to say she'd found the right place to try to begin her medical education. Hobart College, the former Geneva Medical College, received a donation to create a school for women, William Smith College.

In retrospect, Mary Walker seems the most radical of the three women pioneers. Today, the equality she sought for her sex is much more real than it was at her death in 1919. I believe it would be rare today, for example, to have to raise a campaign to return Mary's Congressional Medal of Honor, which had been denied in her lifetime.

These are inspired, inspiring stories, all with strong Central New York connections. It is our pleasure to present them to you.

Dick Case
Post-Standard columnist
Syracuse, New York

Elizabeth Blackwell

In the fullest sense of the word a pioneer

by Mary K. LeClair

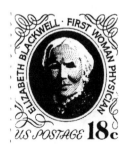

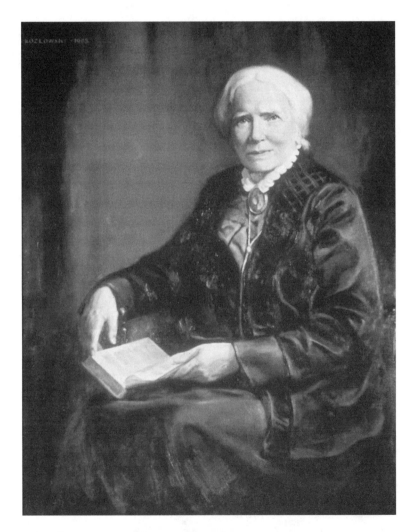

Figure 1: Painting of Elizabeth Blackwell by Joseph Stanley Kozlowski. Painted in 1963. Courtesy SUNY Upstate Medical University.

Previous page: 1974 USPS stamp honoring Dr. Blackwell.

O N JANUARY 23,1849, after many years of determined effort, Elizabeth Blackwell graduated first in her class from Geneva Medical College and became the first woman Doctor of Medicine. Her path to that historic moment was a difficult one, full of obstacles. In the Victorian Age, middle-class women, especially those who married, were only expected to take care of their homes, families, and be subordinate to their husbands. Women did not receive formal educations; they could not own property or vote. Women's options for working outside of the home were limited. It was unorthodox for women to pursue professional careers. Few jobs, such as teaching, were proper for women. Even women teachers were expected to dismiss their careers when they married.

Despite the cultural barriers that were present during the mid-1800s, Elizabeth attended Geneva Medical College and earned an advanced degree. Elizabeth's career in medicine was difficult as she fought to find employment in the male dominated profession of medicine. Hospitals,which were predominately staffed by men, extended no opportunities for Elizabeth to set up a medical practice. There were other cultural forces in place as well. It was not customary for professionals to discuss subjects pertaining to the body, illnesses or

3

diseases in the company of women. Social norms did not call for women to be educated about the human body, its functions, or healthcare.

Unrestrained by these obstacles, Elizabeth's fortitude helped her to become successful as a physician and establish her own medical practice. She founded the New York Infirmary for Women and Children and aided in the creation of its medical college. In England, Elizabeth helped found the National Health Society and was the first woman to be placed on the British Medical Register. Elizabeth is considered a pioneer in the research and development of preventive medicine and a voice of reason and education to women by raising the public's awareness of proper female hygiene in the United States as well as England.

Elizabeth was a nonconformist in her personal life just as she was in her professional career. Elizabeth chose not to marry. The woman's role in marriage was too constraining for Elizabeth. Instead she chose to remain single for her entire life. At mid-age, she adopted an orphan girl and raised her as a single mother.

The Early Years

Born in Bristol, England on February 3, 1821, Elizabeth was the third of nine children of Samuel and Hannah Blackwell, a sugar refiner and his wife. She grew up in the family's home, which was located next door to the refinery, and received her first instruction from a governess. The home was comfortable and beautifully landscaped, with a garden and many trees, flowers and shrubs. The family also enjoyed a vacation summer home, which was about nine miles out of town.

Elizabeth was a perfectionist, stubborn and inquisitive. She had a determined spirit. If there was something she couldn't do—a game she couldn't play, a book she had trouble understanding or a math problem she couldn't solve—she would persist and work at it until she succeeded with the challenge at hand.

Samuel and Hannah Blackwell were devout Methodists. They valued the importance of teaching their children to accept and be accountable for responsibilities. Each morning, along with their servants, the family would read from the Bible and say prayers. On Sundays, the Blackwells would attend church services twice and use the remainder of the day to memorize hymns and biblical passages. The Blackwells were strong supporters of social reform. In England, and later in America, they worked to end slavery and promote suffrage, education reform and equal rights for women. Despite the convention of the time for girls to be quiet, passive, and restrained, her parents encouraged vigorous physical exercise. The children often walked and played outside in their garden. Their governess took them for walks into town and across the countryside.

In 1832, the economy settled into a depression. Further, there was a cholera outbreak so Elizabeth's family decided to emigrate from England to New York. They settled in New York City where Samuel set up a sugar refinery on Congress Street and Elizabeth and her siblings attended school.

Their new life in America was different. The Blackwell family lived in a row house where their rooms were on different floors as if each were stacked on top of the other and the kitchen was in the basement. Their backyard was disproportionately small compared to the house, and they shared a communal water pump with their neighbors. Elizabeth and her two older sisters found great joy investigating their new neighborhood. They walked the streets and observed their new community at work—bankers, grocers and tanners. At times Elizabeth walked up to 18 miles a day curiously exploring her new setting. Before long her younger brother, Sam, who was also gifted with a sense of intellectual curiosity and physical energy, accompanied Elizabeth on her adventures.

As they walked together, they would talk about the books they were reading and share their thoughts about the world.

In addition to their outdoor adventures, the Blackwell children would sing, dance, and play their musical instruments together. The family enjoyed the arts. They frequently attended local concerts and plays.

Unfortunately, the gaiety of their new life in New York would soon diminish. The abolitionist movement was gaining momentum in the United States, and the Blackwells joined in the divisive fight to end slavery. The Blackwell family hid slaves and sympathizers who were being threatened with lynching for speaking out against slavery. The children brought the Abolitionist movement into the schools and echoed their parents' sentiments by speaking out against slavery. They were punished for it. The boys were frequently harassed and often came home with bloody noses and torn clothing. Elizabeth learned that social change came with a price.

By age 15, Elizabeth was attending anti-slavery meetings. Her sister, Anna, was a delegate at anti-slavery conventions and meetings. Involvement in the abolitionist movement and school attendance gave Elizabeth a full life. "As a daily pupil in an excellent school in New York, entering ardently into the anti-slavery struggle, attending meetings and societies, the years passed rapidly away," Elizabeth wrote.

By September 1836, the Blackwells were in dire financial trouble. The economy was failing, and adding to the hardships, her father's refinery caught fire and was destroyed. The refinery was uninsured, and the family's entire investment was lost. In early 1837, the Blackwells did not have enough money to keep their home. The family was forced to dismiss their servants. They survived on a diet of primarily potatoes and earned money by bringing people into their house as paying boarders.

In 1838, Samuel decided to move the family to Cincinnati, Ohio, where he intended to set up the only sugar refinery in the West. At age 17, Elizabeth was the oldest child in the family to make the trip. Her two older sisters, Anna and Marian, had jobs teaching that they could not afford to give up, so they stayed behind.

"We left New York full of hope and eager anticipation," Elizabeth wrote. "We were delighted with the magnificent scenery of the mountains and rivers as we crossed Pennsylvania by canal and stage, and sailed down the noble Ohio River, then lined with forests."

For a few months, the family enjoyed their new life in their new home. They attended a Fourth of July picnic and often attended community lectures. Their new lifestyle soon changed. Hardship would continue for the Blackwells in the West as well. Shortly after they established their new life in Ohio, Elizabeth's father died after a brief bout with bilious fever, leaving his family virtually destitute. At that time, Elizabeth was the only one working in the family. She provided music lessons to children in their neighborhood. Elizabeth sent word to her sisters for help. Together they decided to earn a family income by creating a boarding school. They quickly came to Ohio and helped establish a boarding school for young ladies. Meanwhile, the eldest Blackwell brother took a job working in the Cincinnati courthouse, assisting the mayor. The family managed to survive and maintain a home until the younger siblings were grown.

While operating the boarding school, Elizabeth and her sisters remained active in the local political conventions and public meetings. The girls were known to enjoy singing political songs. "It was a most exciting time," she wrote. "During this long struggle our minds rapidly opened to new views of social and religious duty in the untrammeled social atmosphere of the West."

In 1844, Elizabeth had her first adventure on her own. At the age of 23, she was invited to take charge of a boarding school in western Kentucky, then considered to be a wilderness. The position paid room and board, and a salary of $400. Such a wage was too great to refuse. Elizabeth enthusiastically accepted the new job and ventured to Henderson, Kentucky.

Unfortunately, the excitement of Elizabeth's new found independence stopped abruptly when she arrived to her new job. The people of Henderson were friendly to Elizabeth but she never seemed to fit in. She missed her family and the stimulating culture of New York and Cincinnati, where there were lectures, concerts and political meetings. The little town of Henderson had none of these. Elizabeth was motivated to move on.

Eventually, it was the painful injustice of slavery in Kentucky that caused Elizabeth to leave the position after her first year. "Painful social contrasts constantly forced themselves on my notice," she wrote. "I well remember sitting with my hostess, who was reclining in her rocking chair, on a broad, shaded verandah, on a pleasant Sunday morning, listening to the distant church bells and the rustling of locust trees, when the eldest daughter, a tall, graceful girl, dressed for Sunday, in fresh and floating summer drapery, came into the verandah on her way to church. Just at that moment a shabby, forlorn-looking negro in dirty rags approached the verandah; he was one of the slaves working in the tobacco plantation. His errand was to beg the mistress to let him have a clean shirt on that Sunday morning. The contrast of the two figures, the young lady and the slave, and the sharp reprimand with which his mistress from her rocking chair drove the slave away, left a profound impression on my mind."

By August of that year, when Elizabeth returned from Kentucky, she had learned quite a bit about herself. She now realized her strong sense of fortitude and was determined to make it on her own. Marriage, she thought, was not for her, since she felt she could not devote herself solely to being a wife and mother—what she referred to as a life of servitude. Instead, she spent her time studying German, transcendentalism, metaphysics and music. She attended meetings on abolitionism and women's rights.

During this summer, Elizabeth had a dear friend who was dying from cancer. The friend, Mary Donaldson, asked, "Why don't you study medicine? You like to study and you have intelligence. If I had been treated by a lady doctor, my worst sufferings would have been spared me."

Women received poor health care during the 1800s. Doctors were forbidden from examining private parts of the female body. Donaldson's comments must have weighted on Elizabeth's mind. Elizabeth thought there must be many women who needed female doctors who could prevent or alleviate women's sufferings from illnesses. Inspired by what seemed impossible, she decided to become a doctor.

While back with her family in Cincinnati, Elizabeth's pathway to medicine began. She started talking with and writing to doctors to gather information about the profession. They told her the idea was hopeless—a lady could not endure medical school. The challenge only encouraged her. Elizabeth had her support network in place. She had the support of her family, who knew she would do anything she put her heart and mind into.

Elizabeth continued teaching to raise money for medical school. In 1845, she found a teaching position at a school owned by the Reverend John Dickson in Asheville, North Carolina. Dickson had once been a doctor, and he owned a medical library. Elizabeth utilized the library as an immediate venue to begin studying medicine.

At Dickson's, Elizabeth taught music. In her free time she read every page of the material in the medical library. She loved to study. "My brain is as busy as can be and consequently I am happy," she wrote her mother.

During her time in North Carolina, Elizabeth perform-

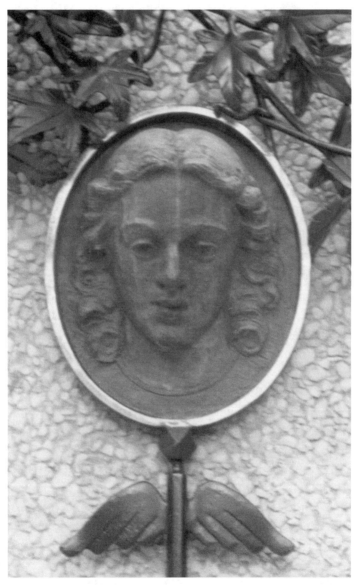

Figure 2: Elizabeth Blackwell sculpture (detail) in Asheville, North Carolina. This sculpture commemorates Blackwell's time in Asheville when she worked as a music teacher prior to attending medical school in upstate New York.   Photo courtesy of Susan Keeter.

ed her first professional medical treatment. Her patient was Miss O'Heara, a friend of the family who had been sick awhile and was being treated with calomel, a mercury compound that commonly made patients throw up and froth at the mouth. One day, Miss O'Heara had a migraine, and Elizabeth utilized hypnotism to cure her migraine.

"I went into her room last night, and found her suffering from an intense throbbing headache. I offered to relieve her, half doubting my own powers, never having attempted anything of the kind; but in a quarter or half an hour she was entirely relieved, and declared some good angel had sent me to her aid," Elizabeth wrote.

Two years later, Elizabeth had enough money saved to begin her search for a medical school. She again started writing to all the doctors she knew and contacted numerous medical schools. Sadly, she received many rejections. Elizabeth was told over and again that medical schools did not admit women, and that patients would not want to be treated by a woman doctor. Some just laughed and told her that men should be doctors and women should be nurses. A few physicians even suggested that she disguise herself as a man in order to gain admittance to a medical school.

"During these fruitless efforts my kindly Quaker adviser, whose private lectures I attended, said to me: 'Elizabeth, it is of no use trying. Thee cannot gain admission to these schools. Thee must go to Paris and don masculine attire to gain the necessary knowledge.' Curiously enough, this suggestion of disguise made by good Dr. Joseph Warrington was also given me by Doctor Pankhurst, the Professor of Surgery in the largest college in Philadelphia. He thoroughly approved of a woman gaining complete medical knowledge; told me that although my public entrance into the classes was out of the question, yet if I would assume masculine attire and enter the college he could entirely rely on two or three of his students to whom he should communicate my disguise, who would watch the class and give me timely notice to withdraw should my disguise be suspected."

Elizabeth wasn't discouraged. She moved to Philadelphia, which at the time was the most popular place to study and practice medicine in America. She rented a room from Dr. William Elder, who became one of several doctors to help her contact medical schools. "He took a generous interest in my plans, helping by his advice and encouragement through the months of effort and refusals which were now encountered," she wrote.

While in Philadelphia she began her studies in anatomy with Dr. Jonathan M. Allen who introduced Elizabeth to the intricate systems in the human body. Elizabeth was fascinated. "With a tact and delicacy for which I have always felt grateful, he gave me as my first lesson in practical anatomy, a demonstration of the human wrist. The beauty of the tendons and exquisite arrangements of this part of the body struck my artistic sense, and appealed to the sentiment of reverence with which this anatomical branch of study was ever afterwards invested in my mind," she wrote.

During the following months, Elizabeth applied for and was denied admission to American medical colleges located predominately in New York City and Philadelphia. Fortunately, a friend, Dr. Warrington suggested that she start applying to smaller medical schools, as they might be more willing to accept her. With Dr. Warrington's help she obtained a list of all the smaller medical schools, called country schools that were located in the northern states. She meticulously examined the prospectus of each school and narrowed her preferences to a group of 12 colleges. The locations selected offered full course loads under esteemed able professors. In the end Elizabeth had applied to a total of 29 American medical colleges.

In November 1847, Elizabeth's perseverance paid off, her dream came true, and she received a letter of admission from Geneva Medical College in Upstate New York, which has since become Hobart and William Smith Colleges. The dean's letter dated October 20, 1847 read:

> *A quorum of the faculty assembled last evening for the first time during the session, and it was thought important to submit your proposal to the class, who have had a meeting this day, and acted entirely on their own behalf, without any interference on the part of the faculty. I send you the result of their deliberation, and need only add that there are no fears but that you can by judicious management, not only "disarm crticism," but elevate yourself without detracting in the least from the dignity of the profession.*

Enclosed with the letter was the following resolution:

> *At a meeting of the entire medical class of Geneva Medical College, held this day, October 20, 1847, the following resolutions were unanimously adopted:*
>
> *1. Resolved—That one of the radical principles of a Republican Government is the universal education of both sexes; that to every branch of scientific education the door should be open equally to all; that the application of Elizabeth Blackwell to become a member of our class meets our entire approbation; and in extending our unanimous invitation we pledge ourselves that no conduct of ours shall cause her to regret her attendance at this institution.*
>
> *2. Resolved—That a copy of these proceedings be signed by the chairman and transmitted to Elizabeth Blackwell.*
>
> *T. J. Stratton, Chairman.*

Geneva Medical College

With a sense of joy and excitement, Elizabeth immediately left Philadelphia traveling night and day to arrive in Geneva two days later. What Elizabeth did not know was that her admission was a point of ridicule and criticism among administrators and students. When Charles Lee, the dean of Geneva Medical College, received Elizabeth's application, it came with a recommendation from Dr. Warrington, an important supporter of the college. Lee didn't want to offend Warrington by not accepting Elizabeth, so he asked the student body to decide if a woman should be admitted. Her admittance was put up to a vote by the students, with few expecting that an almost unanimous vote would occur. One classmate recalled that there was just one dissenter who was cowed by his classmates into voting in favor of Elizabeth's acceptance. Elizabeth would eventually learn that her unanimous acceptance at Geneva Medical College was paradoxically a popular gag rather than a broadly welcomed invitation to study. Many voted to accept her under the notion that it was a joke believing it might have been a hoax initiated by a rival medical school.

Two weeks after agreeing to accept Elizabeth, a diminutive young woman wearing a bonnet that covered her straight blonde hair appeared among them in class. After arriving on campus, Elizabeth immediately signed in, interviewed with the dean and was assigned to her class as student No. 130.

At the end of her first day of classes, she wrote to her mother: "I sit quietly in this large assemblage of young men, and they might be women or mummies for aught I care. I sometimes think I'm too much disciplined, but it is certainly necessary for the position I occupy. I believe the professors don't exactly know in what species of the human family to place me, and the students are a little bewildered."

Initially her attendance drew considerable attention from those in the local community; many came just to watch her take notes in class. After one anatomy class, her teacher offered Elizabeth some help. "You attract too much attention, Miss Blackwell," he told her. "There was a very large number of strangers present this afternoon—I shall guard against this in the future."

Elizabeth was painfully conscious of her effect on the residents of Geneva. "The other people at first regarded me with suspicion but I am so quiet and gentle that suspicion turns to astonishment, even the little boys in the street, stand still and stare as I pass," she wrote. Sometimes this made Elizabeth laugh, sometimes it made her a little sad. Regardless, she came to realize that she was where she needed to be. In a letter to her sister, she wrote, "I cannot but congratulate myself on having found at last the right place for my beginning."

Elizabeth was earnest and worked diligently as a student. Her discipline and dedication helped her to earn the respect and friendship of fellow students. She was respected for her dignified, intelligent, and judicious manner. She referred to the behavior of her fellow classmates as admirable and that of true Christian gentlemen. "[They] fulfilled to the letter the promise contained in their invitation," she said.

Elizabeth was escorted into the classroom by her professors, and she always sat in a seat in the front row. At first, each entrance drew stares, but after only weeks she could enter each class practically unnoticed.

While under the direction of Dr. Le Ford, Elizabeth and four other students were recognized for their exemplary academic performance, and they were privileged to receive an invitation to work with a surgical professor. They toiled many days for long hours that frequently went well into the evening. Students were friendly with Elizabeth, treating her like an older sister and talked freely while in her presence. Her commitment to medical studies grew as did her fascination with the incredible intricacy of the human body.

"Under the intelligent instruction of the demonstrator, anatomy became a most fascinating study. The wonderful arrangements of the human body excited an interest and admiration which simply obliterated the more superficial feelings of repugnance; and I passed hour after hour at night alone in the college, tracing out the ramification of parts, until, suddenly struck by the intense stillness around, I found that it was nearly midnight, and the rest of the little town was asleep," she wrote.

Elizabeth experienced problems in the classroom only once which was during an anatomy class that was slated to discuss the human reproductive systems. Her professor, Dr. Webster, demonstrated obvious reservations about allowing Elizabeth to sit through his lecture. He wrote her and told her that he thought it would be better for her "feminine modesty" if she did not come to class, but instead study the material separately. Elizabeth was indignant—she wanted to receive the same quality of medical education as the men. She responded to the letter in writing. "In this note I told him that I was there as a student with earnest purpose, and as a student simply I should be regarded; that the study of anatomy was a serious one, exciting profound reverence, and the suggestion to absent myself from any lectures seemed to me a grave mistake."

To appease the professor, she offered to sit in the back row and take off her bonnet in order to be less visible. She also said that if her fellow students did not want her to be in class she would forgo her attendance. No matter how important her attendance was, Elizabeth would not go if her presence interfered with the other students learning. Dr. Webster read Elizabeth's note to the class, and they applauded when she joined them. There were no further attempts during her stay in Geneva to shelter her from any aspect of her studies in medicine.

The students at Geneva Medical College inspired Elizabeth to perform well and pursue her dream at having a career in medicine. One day as part of an anatomy lesson, Elizabeth sat in on an examination of a female patient with Dr. Webster. Elizabeth observed that the woman appeared to be humiliated by having to be examined by a man. For Elizabeth, the experience served as an incentive for her to become a doctor. She recognized and identified with the woman's humiliation and reaffirmed that she must become a doctor. "I felt more than ever the necessity of my mission."

Although her academic colleagues grew to accept her, the people living in the community of Geneva did not. Elizabeth had trouble finding a place to live after people in the community discovered she was attending medical school. When Elizabeth strolled out to walk around the town, small boys would stare at her "as a curious animal" and called her names. They treated her as if she was a bad woman or one who was crazy. Women on the streets pulled their skirts aside when they passed her so that their clothing would not touch. Elizabeth endured and eventually found herself a room in a boarding house that was within walking distance from campus. To feel at home, she decorated her room with mementoes from her friends and family. The social acts of rejection caused Elizabeth to want to hurry through the streets and avoid the local people. Even though she was surprised by the poor welcome, she used the rejection and isolation as an opportunity to concentrate on her school work. She spent many nights at school or shut herself in her room to read her books and study her college material.

"I had not the slightest idea of the commotion created by my appearance as a medical student in the little town . . . I afterwards found that I had so shocked Geneva propriety that the theory was fully established either that I was a bad woman, whose designs would gradually become evident, or that, being insane, an outbreak of insanity would soon be apparent."

The news that a woman was attending medical school quickly spread beyond Geneva. *The Boston Medical Journal, The Baltimore Sun*, and other publications reported that 26-year-old Elizabeth was studying medicine. The news inspired the fledgling women's rights movement and encouraged many other women to apply or re-apply to medical school. "A very notable event of the year 1848 was the appearance at the medical lectures of a young woman student named Blackwell. She is a pretty little specimen of the feminine gender," was written in *the Boston Medical Journal. The Baltimore Sun* remarked that she should "confine her practice, when admitted, to diseases of the heart."

Medical college was a challenging period in Elizabeth's life in other ways too. Financially, she had little money and had to go without many of the luxuries that she had become accustomed to in her younger years. She missed the flowers and perfume. Additionally, she was lonesome from being so far from her family. For the first time in her life she spent Christmas and New Year's Day by herself. On Christmas she enjoyed reading letters that her family sent while treating herself to 25 cents worth of raisins and almonds— quite an extravagance.

Elizabeth also faced challenges with academics. When she received her acceptance letter from Geneva Medical College the school year had already begun. She missed several days of coursework that she had to make up. To do so, she studied on weekends, nights and early mornings. She studied every evening and continued to study after the other students went home.

Elizabeth used her life's obstacles as an incentive to work hard. Her perseverance paid off as she excelled in her studies. Meanwhile, as part of the medical program, Elizabeth had to complete clinical work and gain experience working with patients before she could graduate. She returned to Philadelphia with hopes of finding a place to do her clinical work. Once again, she faced disappointment as no hospitals wanted to accept her. Her efforts were further maligned because her professors neglected to write her letters of recommendation as they had promised. Over and over, she was told that the field of medicine was not a place for a lady.

Elizabeth was without money and had to resort to giving music lessons to get by until she was finally offered a position to work at Philadelphia's Blockley Almshouse, a hospital and shelter for the very poorest residents. But even her acceptance had a caveat; she was advised by one of the directors of the Almshouse that she needed to get support from all three political parties who sat on the hospital's supervisory commission. Faced with another obstacle Elizabeth was not deterred and she was accepted to work in what was considered one of the worst hospitals in the city.

"He received me most kindly, but informed me that the institution was so dominated by party feeling that if he, as a Whig, should bring forward my application for admission, it would be inevitably opposed by the two other parties — viz. the Democrats and the Native Americans. He said that my only chance of admission lay in securing the support of each of those parties, without referring in any way to the other rival parties. I accordingly undertook my sole act of lobbying."

Blockley Almshouse hospital was overcrowded, poorly heated, inadequately ventilated, and understaffed.

Elizabeth was assigned to work in the women's syphilitic wing, the worst area of the hospital. The patients did not welcome Elizabeth and the nurses were rude to her. In this wing, the patients laid on the floor and sometimes patients even overflowed into the hall floors. It was at this hospital Elizabeth observed firsthand the awful effects of typhus and syphilis—terrible diseases that caused sores on the body, leading to insanity, and then complete paralysis.

As gruesome and disheartening that pain and suffering can cause, Elizabeth did not become discouraged. In fact, her tenure at Blockley Almshouse proved to be a critical time in her career. While working in the women's ward, she concluded some of the diseases affecting women could be avoided through education. Elizabeth believed women should be educated about health. She reaffirmed her belief in the need for equal treatment for and the essential right for women to be informed and able to make basic decisions about their health. Typhus was the topic of her graduation thesis.

In September 1848, Elizabeth completed her time at Blockley Almshouse and anxiously returned to Geneva Medical College and her friends. "My last evening at Blockley. Here I sit writing by my first fire. How glad I am, to-morrow, to-morrow, I go home to my friends!" Her classmates and landlady welcomed her back and even her relationship with the community seemed to improve slightly. While the local women still did not speak to her, they no longer crossed the streets to avoid her.

Elizabeth worked diligently to complete her course work and study for the final exams which were in a few months. At the end of the final semester, a panel of professors tested Elizabeth on every subject she had studied. She was impressively prepared for each question posed to her. Elizabeth's academic accomplishments were recognized by her classmates who waited outside the exam room. They cheered when she came out and informed them that she passed.

On January 23, 1849, Elizabeth graduated as the top student in her class. The ceremony was well attended. An hour before the ceremony was to begin, the Presbyterian Church where the service was held, was filled to capacity. Her brother Henry who was working in New York at the time attended the ceremony. Dispersed in the seats were some of the ladies of Geneva who previously shunned Elizabeth over the past two years. For that memorable graduation day, Elizabeth bought herself a new outfit and neatly braided her hair. She wanted to present herself with dignity in honor to her family, her college and all women in general. "She was very nicely dressed in her black brocaded silk gown, invisibly green gloves, black silk stockings," her brother wrote.

Even though Dr. Webster urged Elizabeth to participate in the pre-graduation ceremonial march, she refused to march through town as was the custom of graduates before the ceremony. Elizabeth believed processions were unladylike. Instead she arrived in church before her classmates, escorted by her brother. When her classmates arrived one graduate offered her his arm and she processed with her class.

After all the other degrees were handed out, Elizabeth was called to the front of the church by President Benjamin Hale, who congratulated her on her success. He saluted her as *Domina* instead of *Domine*, and conferred the medical degree on her. After receiving her medical degree from President Hale, Elizabeth bowed her head and said, "Sir, I thank you. By the help of the Most High, it shall be the effort of my life to shed honor upon your diploma." The audience burst into applause as Elizabeth became the first woman doctor.

Blackwell Builds Her Career

With a medical degree now in hand, Dr. Blackwell ventured to find a place to practice medicine. Ultimately she wanted to work in a hospital as a surgeon. She knew that setting up a medical practice would not be easy. She anticipated that because she was a woman that she would not be allowed to practice medicine in most hospitals in the United States. So, after a brief visit with her family in Cincinnati, Elizabeth set her sights on Paris, France, one of the great medical centers of the world during the 1800s. She hoped French hospitals would be more open-minded and willing to accept a female physician.

The 28-year-old graduate of Geneva Medical College sailed off on a ship from Boston to Paris. She arrived one week later to her first stop—England. Dr. Blackwell loved returning to her homeland. She visited castles, walked in the gardens and took time to write letters home to her family telling them all about her visit. In Birmingham, a well-connected friend got her an invitation to visit Queens Hospital. Unfortunately Dr. Blackwell was greeted rudely. There was an air of skepticism and negative remarks from medical students and staff. Her welcome was all to reminiscent of her treatment back in the United States. Dr. Blackwell moved throughout England. She traveled to various hospitals, and observed varying attitudes and opinions about female physicians. Some were angry, others curious, and few approving.

"It was just a repetition of old scenes; a few minutes' curiosity and then all went on as usual. The students presented the same mixture of faces as our American ones, wore rather better coats, and seemed quicker in their movements," she wrote.

Dr. Blackwell also sought employment in Greenwich, London and Hampstead where she was treated the same— curiosity at first and then rejection. While touring hospitals, students clamored and pressed to look at the lady surgeon. Students peeked through doors and windows to see her.

While visiting the hospital in Birmingham, Dr. Blackwell was invited to observe a surgeon performing an amputation of a patient's leg without using anesthesia. Dr. Blackwell was not startled or surprised by the procedure. Anesthesia was not commonly used during surgeries.

During this time in Dr. Blackwell's life she found happiness and relaxation through her friends who invited her to parties. She also spent much of her free time touring museums. Her presence as a doctor in England was noticed by many people and she received considerable attention in the press. The British magazine *Punch* welcomed her with a poem called "An M.D. in a Gown." *(below is an excerpt)*

Not always is the warrior male,
    Nor masculine the sailor;
We all know Zaragossa's tale,
    We've heard "Billy Taylor";
But far a nobler heroine, she
    Who won the palm of knowledge,
And took a Medical Degree,
    By study at her College.

They talk about the gentler sex
    Mankind in sickness tending,
And o'er the patient's couch their necks
    Solicitously bending;
But what avails solicitude
    In fever or in phthisic,
If lovely woman's not imbued
    With one idea of physic?

Young ladies all, of every clime,
    Especially of Britain,
Who wholly occupy your time
    In novels or in knitting,
Whose highest skill is but to play,
    Sing, dance, or French to clack well,
Reflect on the example, pray,
    Of excellent Miss Blackwell!

The press, both nationally and internationally, took notice of Dr. Blackwell's accomplishment of becoming the first woman to earn a medical degree. Reactions were neutral, positive, and at times condescending, but a letter in the *Boston Medical and Surgical Journal* of February 21, 1849, flatly condemned "the farce, enacted at the Geneva Medical College." The writer concluded, "As this is the first case of the kind that has been perpetrated either in Europe or America, I hope, for the honor of humanity, that it will be the last." The writer called upon the medical profession "to teach other similar institutions the impropriety of following the example." For the most part, most medical institutions followed the advice.

In May 1849, Dr. Blackwell went on to France with high hopes. She applied to several hospitals and was turned away from them all. She attended brilliant lectures at area medical centers and came to understand why so many American doctors came to Paris to complete their education. She wanted a surgical appointment but was once again met with hostility and rejection.

An article titled "An American Doctoress" that appeared in the *Daily Union* in Washington, D.C. on June 27, 1849 made note of Dr. Blackwell's arrival in Paris. "The lady has quite bewildered the learned faculty, by her diploma, all in due form, authorizing her to dose and bleed and amputate with the best of them. Some of them are certain that Miss Blackwell

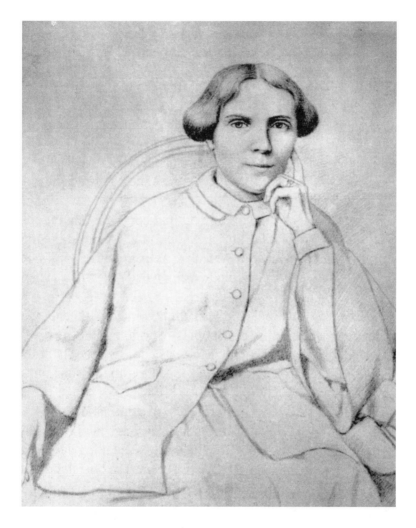

Figure 3: Elizabeth Blackwell, 1859, drawn in Paris by the Comtesse de Charnacee. Courtesy Hobart and William Smith Colleges archives.

is a Socialist of the most furious class, and that her undertaking is the entering wedge to a systematic attack on society by the fair sex."

After about ten days of deliberation on the part of directors of the La Maternité, a government-run maternity hospital that trained midwives, Dr. Blackwell at last received permission to enter the institution as a pupil. Even though she was a licensed physician, the hospital made her enter as an untrained student and work as the other students who were ten years younger than she was and had little or no education. Dr. Blackwell did not let this deter her; she persisted and accepted the job.

Dr. Blackwell worked with patients assisting on operations, helping with births, and attending lectures. Like the other women, she was treated as a servant and not permitted to leave the hospital. Women had no privacy. They slept and bathed in the same area. The food was poor; the schedule was grueling. Dr. Blackwell worked night and day with little sleep delivering babies. She knew the medical material that was being taught. So instead she used the time to learn French memorizing and repeating the lessons until she became proficient in French.

Dr. Blackwell's life would change dramatically in the early morning of November 4, 1849. During her fifth month at the maternity hospital, Dr. Blackwell was taking care of a baby who had a very serious eye infection. The hospital room was dimly lit. As Dr. Blackwell leaned over to irrigate the baby's eye, some spray splashed back into Dr. Blackwell's left eye. Within 12 hours, Dr. Blackwell's eye was swollen and infected. Despite treatment Dr. Blackwell realized that she was going blind from an infection. Within three days the sight in her left eye was gone. She underwent surgery and subsequent treatments but eventually her eye had to be removed to prevent the infection from going to her other eye. Dr. Blackwell had to wear a glass eye for the rest of her life.

"Ah! How dreadful it was," she wrote "to find the daylight gradually fading as my kind doctor bent over me, and removed with exquisite delicacy of touch the films that had formed over the pupil! I could see him for a moment clearly, but the sight soon vanished, and the eye was left in darkness."

Dr. Blackwell knew her vision problems would prevent her from ever being a surgeon. For three weeks following the surgery, she lay in bed in the hospital with both eyes bandaged. She became depressed and her sister, Anna, came to the hospital and took her home to England for the next six months. During that time, she was terribly weak and incapable of reading or writing. Nearly one year later in 1850, Dr. Blackwell regained her strength and ability to study. Despite the glass eye, she was resolved to the fact that she would never be a surgeon but must go on with her life as a doctor.

"Both anatomical and surgical work were out of the question; and even reading had to be laid aside," she wrote.

In October 1850, her spirits were further rejuvenated when she was accepted as a graduate student at St. Bartholomew's Hospital in England. She worked at St.Bartholomew's with Dr. James Paget. It was on this trip that she met with Florence Nightingale. They became friends. Nightingale was a woman who desperately wanted to be a nurse but her parents disapproved of it, saying a hospital was no place for a young lady. Florence and Dr. Blackwell spent much of their time discussing medicine. They believed that healthy living conditions should be practiced and taught by doctors.

"One of my most valued acquaintances was Miss Florence Nightingale, then a young lady at home, but chafing against the restrictions that crippled her active energies. Many an hour we spent by my fireside in Thavies Inn, or walking in the beautiful grounds of Embley, discussing the problem of the present and hopes of the future. To her, chiefly, I owed the awakening to the fact that sanitation is the supreme goal of medicine, its foundation and its crown," Dr. Blackwell wrote.

After a time, when she was 30 years old, Dr. Blackwell grew tired of working as a student in London. She wanted to work as a doctor. She decided to return to America and try to open a practice there. During that time there was hope; life in America was changing for women and efforts were being made to open schools for females. She arrived in New York City with the expectation of finding a place to open a doctor's office. But the landlords did not want a lady doctor in their buildings. Doors were slammed shut on her. Resolute and armed with excellent recommendations, she applied to hospitals, including the women's department of a large City dispensary. Still, all her applications were refused. No one would take her despite all her training.

Ignoring the rejection, Dr. Blackwell decided to open her first practice in the United States in a building on University Place overlooking Washington Square. Her landlady would not allow her to put a sign out that said Elizabeth Blackwell, M.D. so she advertised in the newspaper. She waited for patients but no one came. Dr. Blackwell did not want to wait any longer; she decided to offer health education to women. She organized talks on the physical education of women. She delivered lectures on the physical education for girls in the basement of a Sunday school room in the spring of 1852. Young girls needed exercise, education, fresh air and sunshine, she said.

Dr. Blackwell informed young women about the health risks of wearing corsets. She explained to them how steel corsets that tightened around the waist prevented them from breathing and digesting food properly. The clothing even made it hard for women to walk. Dr. Blackwell also spent her time writing. In 1852, she published the lectures under the title "The Laws of Life in reference to the Physical Education of Girls."

"The first seven years of New York life were years of very difficult, though steady, uphill work. It was carried on without cessation and without change from town, either summer or winter. I took good rooms in University Place, but patients came very slowly to consult me. I had no medical companionship, the profession stood aloof, and society was distrustful of the innovation," Dr. Blackwell wrote.

Dr. Blackwell's lectures on the physical education for girls were attended by a few Quaker women who would later become her first patients. The family of Mr. Stacy B. Collins, a highly respected member of the Society of Friends, was the first family to seek out Dr. Blackwell as their family physician.

"Indeed, my practice during those early years became very much a Quaker practice; and the institutions which sprang up later owed their foundation to the active support of this valuable section of the community," she wrote.

Eventually her medical practice grew, but it grew much too slowly for Dr. Blackwell. She decided to open another office but this time in a poor neighborhood. Three afternoons a week, she saw patients free of charge. It took awhile for patients to start coming to her office but by January 1854 she had a large enough practice to set up a business called the New York Dispensary for Poor Women and Children.

Dr. Blackwell thoroughly enjoyed the work. If patients were too ill to travel she made house calls. She treated their ailments but also gave them information for their minds regarding hygiene, cleanliness and exercise. Some patients were so poor that they could not pay her anything, but many others could. That year she bought a house, and opened a new practice there.

By October 1854, Dr. Blackwell had a busy medical practice. Despite the busyness Dr. Blackwell felt a growing sense of loneliness. She wanted someone to love. She was ready to take another big chance in her life and make a radical decision. She visited a state-run orphanage and adopted an Irish orphan named Katherine "Kitty" Barry.

"The utter loneliness of life became intolerable. . .I took a little orphan girl from the great emigrant depot of Randall's Island to live with me," Dr. Blackwell wrote.

Kitty was a frail seven-year-old girl who brought laughter, warmth, hugs and purpose to Elizabeth's life. They became a family and got a dog, a mastiff named Lion, which they both loved. Dr. Blackwell was very happy. She was full of hope and promise for the future. She now had a busy medical practice and a family.

Dr. Blackwell continued to receive loving support and encouragement from her family. In 1856, her brother Sam and his wife moved into Dr. Blackwell's house in New York and his wife, Nettie, had a baby girl, Florence. Her other family members came from Cincinnati (Henry, Lucy, Mama, and Marian). And from England came Dr. Emily Blackwell. Emily had graduated with honor from the Medical College of Cleveland, Ohio two years earlier (1854) and had been pursuing studies in Europe gaining surgical experience. For a short period the majority of the Blackwells lived together again.

At this time, Dr. Blackwell decided to open a hospital, staffed entirely by women. Yet another daring initiative that would be met with much skepticism.

"This first attempt to establish a hospital conducted entirely by women excited much opposition. At that date, although college instruction was being given to women students in some places, no hospital was anywhere available either for practical instruction or the exercise of the woman-physician's skill," Dr. Blackwell wrote.

The medical staff first consisted of Drs. Elizabeth and Emily Blackwell and Dr. Marie Zakrzewska, an immigrant from Poland whom Elizabeth had encouraged in her medical education. When she started telling people about her plans the feedback was reminiscent of many years ago. "It can't be done," they said. Dr. Blackwell remained determined and asked abolitionist women who organized earlier against slavery to help her raise funds. On May 12, 1857, the New York Infirmary for Indigent Women and Children opened its doors at 64 Bleecker St., a highly respectable area of the city. People from the anti-slavery society, the temperance union and other socially conscious organizations attended the grand opening. The hospital charged $4 a week for those who could afford; others were treated for free. One week's budget came to $22 and included food, wages, heat and lighting. The New York Infirmary was a success, run solely by women, in less than a year treating nearly 1,000 patients.

Having established access to healthcare for women in America as well as a new doorway to help women to work in the medical field, Dr. Blackwell set her sights on England where there were no British women doctors yet. Her journey was well-timed because in 1858, an effort was underway in England to regulate medical professionals throughout the United Kingdom. Governmental legislation created the General Council of Medical Education and Registration, which was an agency that registered practitioners who passed licensing requirements. Once listed on the Register, a doctor could practice anywhere in the United Kingdom. Fortunately for Dr. Blackwell a separate clause provided for the registration of practitioners' foreign degrees.

Sir Benjamin Brodie, a friend of Dr. Blackwell's

from earlier days when she worked at St. Bartholomew, was president of the council. Through some clever maneuverings, primarily by William Shaen, Dr. Blackwell's name was successfully placed on the Register, thereby making her the first officially recognized woman doctor in Great Britain.

Dr. Blackwell did not fully realize how great a triumph it was. Only after her official registration was documented did the Medical Council realize what it had done. As one observer commented at the time, it was a case of Dr. Blackwell's "walking through a door that officials hadn't realized was open." Hastily they slammed it against any further possibility of a woman getting in. The next female physician Elizabeth Garrett had to wait for six years, until 1865, to get admitted. It took another 12 years before any other women were allowed to be entered on Britain's Medical Register.

Over the decades Dr. Blackwell's achievement became more widely appreciated. In 1959 in the February 11 issue of *Scope Weekly* Dr. Annis Gillie said that Dr. Blackwell's admittance had far greater implications for society. "Her achievement was significant not only for women, but as part of the far larger struggle of all those debarred by virtue of creed, as well as class and sex, from the franchise, from the services, and from universal education in England."

In August of 1859 having achieved this great accomplishment of posting a woman's name on the English registry of doctors, Dr. Blackwell returned to New York. All was going well at the Infirmary, the work was expanding rapidly and their private practice was well maintained Dr. Blackwell took up her work, in addition she lectured. She also made plans to create a new medical college and a school of nursing. She was dissatisfied with society's manner of shutting women out of medical education. Dr. Blackwell thought the existing colleges held low standards of training at female medical schools. Women graduating from New York Hospital and Bellevue were as damaging to the professions as they were their patients.

Drs. Elizabeth and Emily Blackwell began to solicit students and raise money. A spacious house at 126 Second Avenue was purchased and adapted as a hospital and dispensary with the capability of also accommodating several students. During this time, Dr. Blackwell lectured and published letters on the necessity of a four-year medical education for women.

In 1861, it would be the anti-slavery movement and the American Civil War that would hold up the establishment of the college. While Dr. Blackwell was disappointed that her efforts would be temporarily halted, she was brought up believing in human freedom and justice. Her life was surrounded by anti-slavery sympathies both in America and England. For these reasons, Dr. Blackwell supported the war. "In the full tide of our medical activity in New York, with a growing private practice and increasing hospital claims, the great catastrophe of civil war overwhelmed the country and dominated every other interest," she wrote.

At the outbreak of the war, Dr. Blackwell recognized there was a shortage of nurses. She called an informal meeting of the lady managers at the infirmary to see what could be done to help supply trained nurses to the battlefield. Dr. Blackwell intended the meeting to be held in private but Henry Raymond announced it in his paper the "New York Times" and women from the Infirmary and the general public volunteered for training. There were too many for the staff to train and the United States Sanitary Aid Commission and the Women's Central Relief Association was subsequently formed to administer the effort.

Dr. Blackwell served as chair of the registration committee and interviewed and screened candidates. She did not accept women under 30 years of age. The women trained by the Blackwell sisters proved themselves competent and compassionate.

In July 1863 as the war continued, riots broke out after a draft was enacted. Dr. Blackwell and Kitty, now 17, were faced with protecting the Blackwell Infirmary from angry rioters who wanted Dr. Blackwell to remove Black patients from the infirmary. The mob armed with anything from pistols to pitchforks smashed and set fire to other sympathizers homes and businesses. They stoned and hanged Black people in the streets. Dr. Blackwell was resolute and to the surprise of many, the hospital was spared. She carried on caring for her patients in spite of the critics who knew of Blackwell's sympathies against slavery.

After the war, the Infirmary was very busy and Dr. Blackwell went back to devoting her efforts to establishing a medical college for women. In November 1868, the Woman's Medical College of the New York Infirmary opened. Its earliest lectures were delivered from rented space in what is now part of New York University. At the women's college, Dr. Blackwell set very high standards for admission, academic and clinical training, and certification for the school. Three women served on its faculty: Emily Blackwell was professor of obstetrics and diseases of women; Lucy Abbott was her assistant and taught clinical midwifery and Elizabeth was a professor of hygiene becoming the first professor of preventive medicine in America.

In 1869, at the age of 48 and 20 years since she graduated as the first woman physician, the public recognition of the women physicians had grown. In the northern states the free and equal entrance of women into the profession of medicine had been secured. In Boston, New York and Philadelphia special medical schools for women were designated by the government, and in some long established colleges women were received as students in ordinary classes. Dr. Blackwell was satisfied with the progress and returned home to England by the time the first class graduated from the Woman's Medical College.

"Our New York center was well organized under able guidance, and I determined to return to England for a temporary though prolonged residence, both to renew physical strength, which had been severely tried, and to enlarge my experience of life, as well as assist in the pioneer work so bravely commencing in London," Dr. Blackwell wrote.

In London, she did not rest. Dr. Blackwell set up a medical practice and taught at the London School of Medicine for Women. She gave lectures at the Working Women's College addressing subjects such as "How to Keep a Household in Health."

In 1871, Dr. Blackwell achieved yet another first. She was invited to attend a small meeting in the drawing room of 6 Burwood Place in London to consider the subject of establishing a means to educate the public on sanitary issues. There the National Health Society was formed with the motto "Prevention is better than cure." A few years later when the London School of Medicine for Women was established Dr. Blackwell accepted the position as chair of gynecology in the college.

In 1879, Dr. Blackwell moved to Hastings and spent many years writing. She authored "Counsel to Parents on the Moral Education of Their Children" an outspoken book on sex education. She sent the manuscript to 12 of the leading London publishers, who all declined the publication. Dr. Blackwell printed a small edition herself which one bookseller agreed to sell. She also wrote in opposition of using animals in scientific medical experiments.

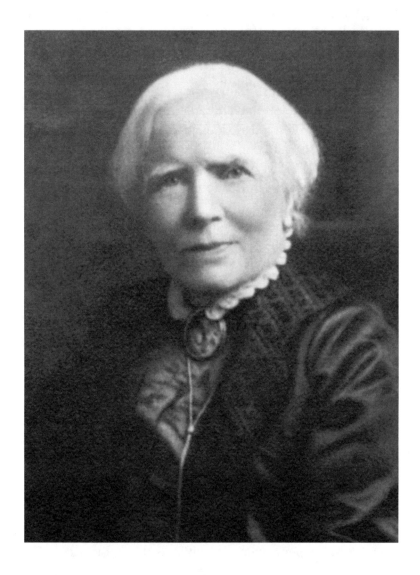

Figure 4: Detail of Blackwell portrait (fig. 1, p. 2)

Throughout the 1880s Dr. Blackwell continued writing, publishing three books in three years—*Christian Socialism, Wrong and Right Methods of Dealing with the Social Evil*, and *The Human Element in Sex*. She also continued to travel. In 1889, she lectured in Paris and in 1897 she addressed a forum of physicians in London concerning the health of the Army in India.

In the end, she sought to counsel physicians on their duties to society and to encourage female physicians to carry out her life's ambition.

"It has become clear to me that our medical profession has not yet fully realized the special and weighty responsibility which rests upon it to watch over the cradle of the race; to see that human beings are well born, well nourished, and well educated. The onward impulse to this great work would seem to be especially incumbent upon women physicians, who for the first time are beginning to realize the all-important character of parentage in its influence upon the adult as well as on the child—i.e. on the race," Dr. Blackwell wrote.

She also remained adamant for equality and cooperation between genders, while always maintaining the religious beliefs that her parents instilled in her as a young child. "The study of human nature by women as well as men commences that new and hopeful era of the intelligent co-operation of the sexes through which alone real progress can be attained and secured. We may look forward with hope to the future influence of Christian women physicians when, with sympathy and reverence guiding intellectual activity, they learn to apply the vital principles of their Great Master to every method and practice of the healing art," she wrote.

Throughout the 1890s the New York Infirmary carried on its ever increasing work. A nurses' training school was started in 1894 and in 1897 a fire burnt down the medical college section of the building. By 1899 Cornell University absorbed the college as there was no need for a separate college for women.

In 1907, Dr. Blackwell fell down a flight of stairs at a hotel and never fully recovered. Before dying she would receive good news. Dr. Blackwell learned that William Smith of Geneva gave Hobart College, the former Geneva Medical College, almost $500,000 to endow a school for women— William Smith College. The college used Smith's donation to erect a hall of science in which biological and psychological laboratories were established.

On May 31, 1910, the great pioneer woman of medicine died in England at the age of 89. Her obituary said, "She was in the fullest sense of the word a pioneer, who like all pioneers, heard but did not listen." Kitty buried her in Scotland.

The epitaph on her grave reads:

"In loving memory of Elizabeth Blackwell, M.D., born at Bristol 3rd February, 1821, died Hastings 31st May, 1910.

The first woman of modem times to graduate in medicine (1849) and the first to be placed on the British Medical Register (1859).

It is only when we have learned to recognize that God's law for the human body is as sacred as—nay, is one with— God's law for the human soul that we shall begin to understand the religion of the heart."

"Love seeketh not her own" (I Cor. Xiii, 5)
"The pure in heart shall see God" (Matt. v. 8).

The Blackwell Legacy

As a reminder and tribute to Dr. Blackwell, her portrait hangs in the London School of Medicine for

Women and also in the Blackwell House at Hobart and William Smith Colleges. In 1906, the first women's dormitory on the Geneva campus was named in her honor.

In 1974 Dr. Blackwell was honored on an 18-cent United States Postage Stamp, commemorating the 125th anniversary of her graduation. In 1975, the Elizabeth Blackwell Health Center for Women was founded in Philadelphia.

Today, in her honor, the Elizabeth Blackwell Award is given by Hobart and William Smith Colleges to a woman whose life exemplifies outstanding service to humanity. In 1994, a full-sized sculpture, created by Professor of Art A.E. Ted Aub, was placed at the center of the campus. Engraved in the sculpture's granite base is an excerpt from a letter Blackwell wrote from Geneva in 1847: "I cannot but congratulate myself on having found at last the right place for my beginning."

Bibliography

Abram, Ruth J. *Women Doctors in America, 1835-1920*. New York: W. W. Norton & Company, 1985.

Blackwell, Elizabeth. *Pioneer Work in Opening the Medical Profession to Women*. London: J.M. Dent & Sons, LTD. New York: E.P. Dutton & Co., (exact date unknown, first edition, 1895). Introduction by Milicent G. Fawcett.

Chambers, Peggy. *A Doctor Alone*. London: The Bodley Head, 1956.

Sahli, Nancy Ann. *Elizabeth Blackwell, M.D*. New York: Arno Press, 1982.

Smith, Warren Hunting. *Hobart and William Smith: The History of Two Colleges*. Geneva: Hobart and William Smith Colleges, 1972.

Wilson, Dorothy Clarke. *Lone Woman: The Story of Elizabeth Blackwell The First Woman Doctor*. Boston: Little, Brown and Company, 1970.

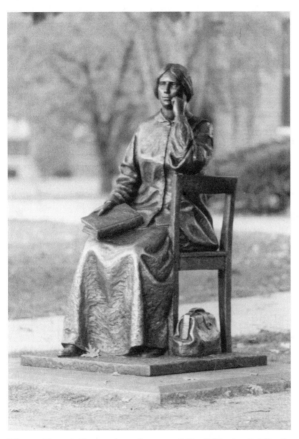

Figure 5: A full-sized sculpture of Dr. Elizabeth Blackwell, created by Professor of Art A.E. Ted Aub, sits on the Quadrangle at Hobart and William Smith Colleges in Geneva, New York.

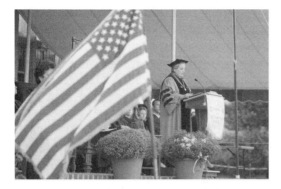

Figure 6: Former Secretary of State Madeleine Albright in the 2001 Ceremony of Hobart and William Smith Colleges where she received the Elizabeth Blackwell Award. Photo courtesy of Hobart and William Smith Colleges.

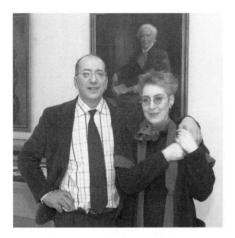

Figure 7: Elizabeth Blackwell day is an annual celebration at SUNY Upstate Medical University in Syracuse, New York. The 2006 keynote address was delivered by Brian Hurwitz, MD, Kings College, London and Ruth Richardson, DPhil, of the University of Cambridge. Photo courtesy of SUNY Upstate Medical University.

Dr. Mary Walker

"A Missionary Spirit"

by Justin D. White
Oswego Town Historian

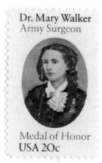

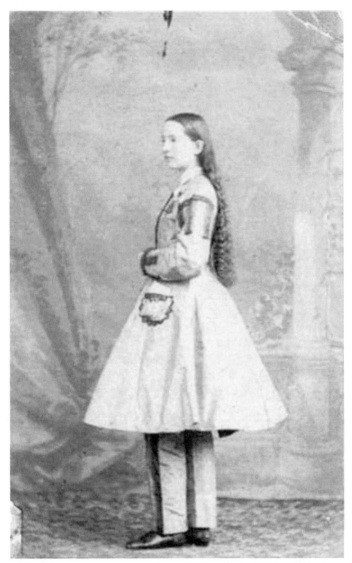

Figure 8: This photograph of Dr. Mary Walker was taken in London, England during her lecture tour between 1866-1867. Mary is seen here in a light-colored bloomer costume with embroidered details and matching pants beneath. This outfit, along with her waist long hair, shows that Mary's fashion sense was still feminine well after the end of the Civil War. It appears that she is also wearing her Medal of Honor proudly. Courtesy of the Oswego County Historical Society Collections.

Previous page: USPS stamp issued in 1982 to honor Dr. Walker.

"Society pays a premium to women for being deceitful, by being sure to abuse those who dare to be honest and frank."

~ Mary E. Walker, M.D. (1832-1919), *HIT*, 1871

L ONG BEFORE DR. MARY EDWARDS WALKER became the first and only woman ever awarded the nation's highest military honor, the Congressional Medal of Honor, and reached the heights of national fame, she was a crusader for human rights and equality. Mary was once described by a peer as having a "missionary spirit; the desire to do good...and the desire to do right under all circumstances." [1] Mary's undeniable determination to have equal rights under the law for all women, and to live in the way she chose, was a basic will that would carry her through life. Long after her death, Mary's personal thoughts survive today in the written word and remain as a testament to her beliefs; words that still ring true today:

"God has given to woman just as defined and important gifts of individuality, as He has to man; and any man-made laws that deprive her of any rights or privileges, that are enjoyed by himself, are usurpations of power...for her

45

aspirations and freedom of soul, are as dear to her as is her life," Mary wrote. "Deity intended a free and full development of all of woman's powers, as well as man's, and gave her a mind to decide for herself all things." [2]

These are the powerful and effective words of Dr. Mary E. Walker: a physician, Medal of Honor recipient, women's rights leader, dress reform crusader, philosopher, writer and beyond. When reviewing her life, it could easily be said that Mary was a woman who lived a century before her time. She blazed a trail that still burns bright. The path she left behind leads to an amazing journey through trial and triumph, honor and defeat, and celebrity and poverty.

The same struggles in modern day movements are the ones that she forged, only to be forgotten and remembered again a century later. Mary's dreams and desires, seemingly simple by modern standards, were mainly unacceptable by the majority view in 19th-century America. She boldly refused to yield to conventional, psychological and physical Victorian constraints. During Mary's lifetime her words and actions were outrageously radical.

The Early Years

It was in the year 1832 that Mary's parents Alvah and Vesta (Whitcomb) Walker settled in the small, rural countryside of the town of Oswego in upstate New York. It was there Alvah purchased a 33-acre farm on a rural country road called Bunker Hill. A modest and comfortable wooden farmhouse was built on the site, nearly five miles from the small, but thriving village of Oswego. The village later became the port city of the same name, situated along the great shores of Lake Ontario. The area along the waterways was growing at a rapid pace. The Oswego River and Lake Ontario provided excellent resources for economic opportunities, and the community eventually was built around the power of the river and lake. The advantages seemed endless and possibilities flourished with trade from Canada.

When Alvah Walker moved his family to the area, he soon established a livelihood as a farmer on the land. At the time the Walker's settled in Oswego, their young family included four daughters: Aurora, Vesta, Luna and Cynthia. Mother Vesta was soon expecting another child upon their arrival in Oswego. The Walkers could never have predicted that their fifth daughter, Mary, born November 26, 1832, would become a national sensation and perhaps the most legendary of Oswego's citizens.

Named for her paternal aunt, the seemingly common name was a departure from the more unique and unusual names the Walkers had chosen for their other children. Mary, however ordinary in name, was destined to live an extraordinary life. She would grow up to be a woman steadfast in her convictions. Mary's undying devotion to her beliefs, especially those of women's rights and equality, were a product of her early family life. The environment in which she was raised was unlike that of other middle-class girls of the era. It was primarily Mary's father and his personal philosophies on education, health and hygiene that held such a huge impact on her life.

Mary's biographer Dr. Charles M. Snyder wrote, "Mary's home reflected the convictions of her much-traveled father. One of the less orthodox of these was that girls should be educated, and encouraged to pursue professional careers ... He believed, also, that their health should not be impaired by tight-fitting clothing." [3]

Mary herself once said in an interview, "From a very young girl I had strict ideas in regard to dress. My father had studied medicine and we were taught very early the laws of hygiene. He forbade us to wear corsets...I have never worn them. No, sir, my waist has never been confined in one of those steel traps; it is just as nature intended it should be—free and unconfined." [4] The fact that none of the Walker daughters wore corsets was a complete departure from the acceptable female dress code of the era.

In 1833, the last Walker child was born, a boy named Alvah, Jr. "Like their brother, the Walker daughters were encouraged in their intellectual pursuits even as they were required to participate fully in the arduous chores of farm life. This early experience of equal treatment from her family shaped Walker's ambitions and her irrepressible determination to demand the same from the world beyond her door," [5] wrote biographer Elizabeth Leonard. Yet, the conservative world beyond the isolated Walker farm would not espouse the same views as Mary or her family.

Education

It was in the Bunker Hill schoolhouse, built by her father, where Mary received her primary education. When she was eighteen she followed the footsteps of her older sisters and attended Falley Seminary in the nearby community of Fulton, New York. Her coursework consisted of the basic classes of algebra, natural philosophy, grammar and "surprisingly for a young woman, physiology and hygiene." [6]

She left Falley Seminary in 1852 to pursue one of the few acceptable and respectable careers for a young lady—teaching. Yet, Mary always wanted to go beyond the boundaries her gender held for her. She soon left the one-room country school and set her sights on a nearly impossible goal for a woman in the midst of 19th-century America: to be a female physician.

From a young age, Mary always challenged conventional ideas; especially when they held her back. After all, this was a time of radical change. Abolitionism, temperance, women's rights and other radical movements, including a Utopian society, were all brewing at this time in Central New York. A few years earlier, in 1848, the first Women's Rights Convention had met in Seneca Falls, New York. In the same year, John Humphrey Noyes established a communal colony in Oneida, New York. In 1849, Elizabeth Blackwell beat the odds and became the first woman physician in America. Meanwhile, abolitionists across the state were pushing the cause for antislavery. Brave men and women were harboring fugitives, assisting in escapes to Canada and fighting for human rights.

Perhaps the biggest of these impressions on 16-year-old Mary was the graduation of Blackwell from Geneva Medical College. Mary had been educated well by her family and it appears she was not afraid to try new things. Blackwell's accomplishment probably further inspired her belief that she too could achieve anything she put her mind to; but probably no one, including her family, could foresee how far she was prepared to go.

In a bold move, she applied and was accepted as a medical student at the eclectic Syracuse Medical College in Syracuse, New York. Eclecticism was a far less conventional form of medical training, typically drawing from a variety of methods and styles. The theories of eclectic training were often unaccepted in the mainstream medical community. After two years of study, Mary received her diploma in June of 1855. At age 21, and the only woman in her graduating class, Mary had a medical degree and became one of the select few female physicians in the United States. [7]

Mary was one of two speakers at her class graduation. On that day she said, "As graduates we are soon to leave and perform the active duties of the profession, and we trust you will never be pained by hearing that any have failed to be successful in, and respected by the community where we may chance to reside."[8] Sadly, Mary's idealistic words on her graduation day would not include her. Not only had she received untraditional training, she would also be forced over and over to prove herself in what was considered a male profession.

Snyder wrote, "In retrospect, it would appear that Mary's bid for acceptance by the public was doomed from the start. The prejudice facing any female physician was a formidable handicap." [9]

The other speaker at Mary's graduation was Dr. Albert Miller, "recognized as a gifted scholar and orator." His graduation speech addressed the ideas of the "The True Thinker," and preached of the eclectic, free thinker ideas that Syracuse Medical College promoted. [10] Miller was more than just a fellow student, he was also an admirer of Mary's. The feeling was mutual and Mary accepted Miller's proposal of marriage.

Love & Marriage

Shortly after graduation the two were married on November 19, 1855 at the Walker farm in Oswego. As would become her trademark, Mary would flaunt tradition. The Walker—Miller nuptials must have been the most unusual ever witnessed in the lifetime of those in attendance. It has been reported that Mary refused to use the words "obey" in her vows, refused to take her husband's surname in place of her own and refused to wear a traditional wedding dress. Instead, she reputedly wore a version of the scandalous "bloomer" costume.

Mary also asked a Unitarian theologian, the Rev. Samuel J. May of Syracuse, to be the officiator of the ceremony. Reverend May was a staunch abolitionist, prolific writer and public speaker, well known throughout Central New York for his own outspoken ideas. [11] The wedding was chronicled in local newspapers, including reports in Oswego and Syracuse:

"The old proverb that two of a grade can not agree has some exceptions, truly. In the (Syracuse) *Chronicle* to-day, appears the rare announcement of the marriage of two doctors, bona fide M.D.'s, viz: Albert E. Miller, M.D., of Rome, and Mary E. Walker, M.D., of Oswego town. Thus paired the two established themselves in Rome, and commenced business under the firm of Dr. Miller & Miller Walker, the wife still retaining an identity of her own in the business affairs by making use of her maiden name. 'If the Doctors are agreed let others hold their peace.'" [12]

Mary wrote this about the occasion: "The noble Rev. Mr. May would not stoop to such a despicable meanness as to ask a woman to 'serve' or 'obey' a man. How barbarous the very idea of one equal promising to be the slave of another, instead of both entering life's greatest drama as intelligent equal parties. Our promises were such as denoted, two intelligent beings instead of one intelligence and one chained." [13]

Mary and Albert settled in Rome, New York following their marriage and she set up a joint practice with her husband. Another biographer, Elizabeth Leonard, wrote, "To focus only on Walker's nonconformism, however, is to forget that she was in many ways also a child of mid-century Victorian culture, a woman who, for example, although she challenged conventions by attending medical school, acquiesced to convention by falling in love ... " [14]

While many of Mary's ideas on marriage, especially the ceremonial aspects, were radical for the times, she also held on to the more traditional values of marriage. She once wrote, "True conjugal companionship is the greatest blessing of which mortals can conceive in this life—to know that there is supreme interest in one individual, and that it is reciprocated." She also believed, "There can be nothing more beautiful, than the true marriages that are so rare ... where soul reads soul, appreciatingly, and neither tries to deceive the other. Such, and such alone, are truly married, and must recognize and practice the great and beautiful laws of true marriage." [15]

Regardless of these ideals, her marriage to Dr. Miller did not last. The two were separated after a short time when revelations of Dr. Miller's infidelity came to light. This was a devastating blow for Mary and was to be her only documented relationship. It is here that Mary's disappointment and distrust of the opposite gender began to develop. While she refused to specifically discuss the subject of her own marriage, she continued to have strong views on the subject of love.

It can be interpreted through her written words how she truly felt about this dark period in her life. "We have often heard it said that men always love women, and are their natural protectors, because of their great strength and great love," she wrote. "Some men love women as children love dolls, and as a natural result, treat them just as dolls are cared for. They dress them in all the finery they are able to procure, pet and exhibit them until the clothes become old, and the beautiful color of the face is gone, and the eyes are contracted and dim, and then, like worn out dolls, they are thrown aside for neighbor's dolls, or for some beautiful images in the show windows of society's false market." [16]

If necessary, Mary also firmly believed in taking action for divorce. "To be deprived of a Divorce is like being shut up in a prison because some one attempted to kill you. The wicked one takes his ease and continues his course, and you take the slanders, without the power to defend yourself." [17] She eventually obtained a divorce from Dr. Miller, an unusual occurrence in the mid-19th century. Not only was divorce rare, it was considered an unacceptable course of action and held a stigma of disgrace.

For Mary, however, the disgrace would have been to stay with a man who mistreated the vows she held sacred. "If it is right to be legally married, it is right to be legally Divorced," she wrote. "Thanks to an increasing and diffusing sentiment of equity that the breezes of time are fast fanning out such unjust ideas as the right of compelling people to live together when that relation is perfectly agonizing ... " [18] After one battle was over, she moved on and preferred to think of her goals and the future. In a very short time she put the past behind her, and Dr. Albert Miller with it.

Mary refocused her energies on her premarital ideas. It was while she was in medical school that she began to experiment with women's clothing. This would soon become one of the primary concerns of her life. Mary firmly believed that the conventional dress of the mid-19th century was detrimental to women's health. She wrote passionately about the subject of dress reform. "The greatest sorrows from which women suffer today are those physical, moral, and mental ones, that are caused by their unhygienic manner of dressing," she wrote. [19] She eventually adopted the bloomer costume, also known as the American Reform Dress. The creation of the style is attributed to Amelia Jenks Bloomer, which consisted of a coat dress that reached below the knees with pants beneath. The style gained popularity among the women's rights advocates, but soon was seen as a distraction due to the negative attention it caused. Mary continued to model the bloomer costume long after it ceased to be a fad. However, a more important issue would interrupt all of Mary plans of the future — at least temporarily.

The Civil War

In 1861, shortly after Mary's failed marriage, her strong patriotic devotion called her attention to the great American Civil War. She expressed her patriotism throughout her life. After

reading a poem she wrote following the war, it is easy to see
why she so much wanted to be a part of the Union cause:

> I love it! I love it! Oh, who shall dare
> To chide me for loving that flag so fair?
> I treasured it long for the patriot's pride
> And wept for the heroes who for it died
> When I am buried 'neath the ground,
> Wrap that flag my corpse around,
> Plant that flag above my grave,
> There let it wave! Let it wave! [20]

Mary headed straight to Washington, D.C., determined
to become involved in the Union cause. "Apparently, without consideration or concern for the opposition she would
engender, Walker headed for the Capital with more than one
letter of recommendation in hand. In Washington, she
promptly began her unprecedented pursuit of an official commission as a surgeon in the Union Army," wrote Leonard. [21]
Her request would be repeatedly rejected.

However, she did not relent and volunteered as an assistant surgeon in a temporary hospital set up in the United States
Patent Office. At first any pair of hands that could help would
do, and officials in charge temporarily overlooked the fact
that she was a woman doctor. As time went on, more and
more people noticed her differences. This would not deter
Mary from doing her part in the war effort. From there she
traveled to the bloodiest battlefields to assist in anyway pos-
sible.

In 1862, she traveled to Warrentown, Virginia to attend to the victims of the Battle of Antietam. One of the bloodiest battles of the war, the Union troops alone suffered more
than 13,000 causalities. Mary arrived ready to help only to
realize there was little she could do to care for the sick and
wounded without clean water and the most basic supplies.

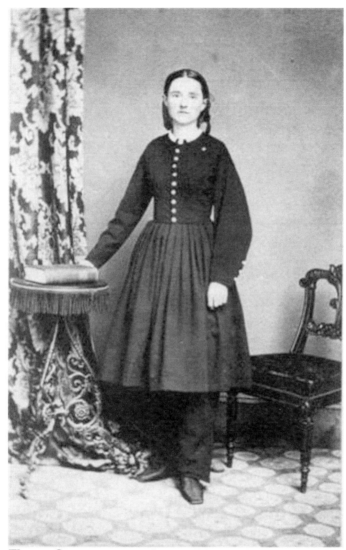

Figure 9: This photograph of Dr. Mary Walker was taken during the Civil War while Mary was in Washington, D.C. This is a very basic bloomer dress with a lace collar and pants beneath. Her long hair is gathered in a snood with tassels, typical of the period. She is wearing a pin at the collar that signified that she was an assistant surgeon. Courtesy of the Oswego County Historical Society Collections.

After struggling to provide some relief, she implored the officials in charge to transport the soldiers that were the most severely wounded to Washington. Mary knew that was the only way she could provide the supplies and facilities necessary. Mary made a convincing argument and General Ambrose Burnside personally requested that Mary escort the soldiers by train to Washington.[22]

In December of 1862, Mary found herself in the midst of history again when she embarked to the fields of Fredericksburg, which had been another devastating battle in the history of the war. A tent hospital was set up where Mary worked again for nothing but rations and a tent to sleep in. During this chaotic time she managed to have a uniform made in the bloomer fashion that strongly resembled that of a union officer, complete with gold buttons. She also wore a green sash about her waist, which had been a signature feature of an army surgeon. Mary surely knew that she had no permission to do so. [23]

By 1863, Mary had seen first hand the tragedy and despair caused by the war. She was haunted by the desperation of hundreds of women and children roaming the streets of Washington, D.C. in search of husbands, fathers and brothers. In an effort to bring families together, Mary established a boarding house in Washington for women looking for their loved ones among the thousands of sick and wounded soldiers. She later extended this project into a second home. She helped to develop the Women's Relief Association, which was established for the benefit of those families traveling to Washington. After seeing so many lost and hopeless women, Mary even placed an ad in a Washington newspaper that read: "Dr. Mary Walker has the pleasure to inform those females who are homeless that she has secured respectable rooms where they can remain overnight, free of charge." [24]

Even through all her volunteer efforts, Mary still wanted to be officially involved with the war effort and recognized with an appointment. With her usual take charge approach, she wrote to President Abraham Lincoln. Her letter was written in the third person and dated January 1864. Mary ended the note to the President by stating, " She will not shrink from duties under shot and shells, believing that her life is of no value in the country's greatest peril if by its loss the interests of future generations shall be promoted." Surprisingly, the President responded to Mary's letter personally, but she failed to persuade him to intercede. In his brief reply the President wrote, "The Medical Department of the army is an organized system in the hands of men supposed to be learned in that profession and I am sure it would injure the service for me, with strong hand, to thrust among them anyone, male or female, against their consent." [25]

Even the gentle let down of the most powerful man in America did not stop Mary from pursuing her official commission. She soon gained the support of other high status officials such as Surgeon General R.C. Wood, General George C. Thomas and even Major General William T. Sherman. Finally, after two years of dedicated service to the union cause, she was given a commission as a civilian contract surgeon, her official title being Acting Assistant Surgeon. This was the status of all civilian surgeons who were also given the military equivalence of First Lieutenant. She remained the only woman to serve as an assistant surgeon in the American Civil War. [26]

Her personal battle would not end here, nor for the rest of her life. "Like most of the 5,500 civilian doctors who ultimately spent time as noncommissioned army contract surgeons, Walker faced a precontact examination of her medical abilities by a board of doctors selected by the Medical Department," wrote Leonard. [27] It seems from the beginning she faced prejudice and when she finally had a chance to become legitimate in the eyes of the government, she was again deceived.

One of the members of the review board called the idea of giving her a contract "absurdity." To him she was a "medical monstrosity ... dressed in that hybrid costume." He further believed, "She had never been...within the walls of a medical college or hospital, for the purpose of obtaining a medical education." [28] As Leonard so aptly points out, Mary would gladly have displayed her diploma for the whole medical board to admire. However, the board did find: "As a nurse, in a general hospital the Board believes her services may be of value and respectfully recommended her for that position." [29] This was an unacceptable consolation prize for Mary.

The board, composed of men of the medical profession, probably did not take kindly in having to examine Mary in the first place. The pre-existing bias toward female physicians may have tainted their decision. The fact that she wore pants may have pushed the issue right over the edge. Surprisingly, the examining board failed to convince Surgeon General Wood and General Thomas that she was incompetent. Her commission was upheld. Mary finally had a taste of victory.

She was assigned as the assistant surgeon of the 52nd Ohio Volunteers, and resentment towards her continued. The regiment's chaplain, the Rev. Nixon Stewart, later included Mary in his memoirs of the war: "She wore curls, so that everybody would know she was a woman," he wrote. "The men seemed to hate her and she did little or nothing for the sick of the regiment." [30] According to Leonard, this may not be far from the truth for there were very few ill soldiers while Mary served the regiment.

Instead she spent most of her time caring for the sick civilians in the surrounding countryside of the camp. The chaplain also wrote, "We thought of our mothers and sisters as our dearest friends," he wrote, " and could not bear the thought of having them share with us the rude usages of camp life. We believed she [Walker] was honest and sincere in her

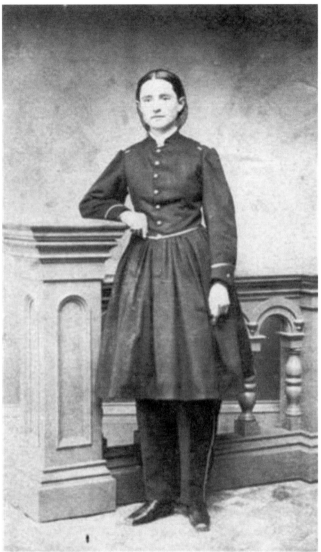

Figure 10: Mary undoubtedly commissioned a seamstress to create this very rare version of the bloomer costume. The outfit is a clear interpretation of the Union army's uniforms and similar to what a civilian surgeon would have worn. Notice the shoulder straps, buttons, braided details and stripe on the pants. This photograph was taken in the Austen Gallery in the city of Oswego, probably just before the end of the Civil War as Mary is not wearing her Medal of Honor. Courtesy of the Oswego County Historical Society Collections.

views ... yet the majority of the men in the regiment thought she was out of her place in the army ... "[31] For the rest of her life, it would not only be soldiers who thought Mary was "out of her place."

In fact, many thought Mary was just a "pretty face" who went way beyond the 19th-century gender boundaries. A reporter captured the story of her unusual services in a local newspaper and conveyed this thought about Mary to readers: "The young lady is very pretty and is said to thoroughly understand her profession. We imagine that the bitter pills which the sick ... take hereafter, will be deprived of a great proportion of their nausea by the fair hands which prescribed them." [32]

In April of 1864, after traveling the countryside alone seeking to help local civilians in need of medical attention she wandered into enemy territory near Chattanooga, Tennessee. She was confronted by a confederate soldier and taken as a prisoner of war just two months after her commission. She was transported to Richmond, Virginia to serve four months in a confederate prison called Castle Thunder. Upon her arrival there was much confusion as to her gender, her profession as a doctor and the exact nature of her military status. Was she a doctor, soldier or spy? Confederate Captain Benedict J. Semmes described the day she arrived at the prison:

"This morning we were all amused and disgusted too at the sight of a *thing* that nothing but the debased and depraved Yankee nation could produce — 'a female doctor' — ... brought in by the pickets this morning. She was dressed in the full uniform of a Federal Surgeon, looks hat & all, & wore a cloak ... and of course had a tongue enough for a regiment of men. I was in hopes the General would have had her dressed in a homespun frock and bonnet and sent back to the Yankee lines, or put in a lunatic asylum ... " [33]

Dr. Mary later made a statement in a lecture she gave

on her Civil War experiences, which almost seems a rhetorical response to this:

"What if such are slandered by those who have not the moral courage to step outside of time-honored customs, when our nation is in peril?" [34]

Varying accounts of prison life range from adequate to poor. Mary stated that the prison was vermin infested and rats roamed freely. The food was fine, she thought, but only two meals a day were served. However, her eyesight was weakened by the poor nutrition, and like other prisoners, she lost a significant amount of weight. Mary's imprisonment did not affect her ability to once again fight for human rights and dignity. In prison, she demanded better food, living conditions and even medical supplies for all inmates. Her captors also had a common request—that she wear clothes "more becoming her sex." [35]

Biographer Elizabeth Leonard wrote, "Those who may have believed that at Castle Thunder Prison she had gotten what she deserved for overstepping the bounds of her gender, and may have expected her time there to have convinced her of the wrongheadedness of pursuing a career in the military, would soon discover that they had given her too little credit and had underestimated the strength of her resolve and her sense of purpose." [36]

Indeed, after her release from prison she went back to Washington for reassignment. She was then commissioned as Acting Assistant Surgeon of the Women's Prison Hospital in Louisville, Kentucky, and later appointed head of an orphan asylum at Clarksville. The greatest conflict America had ever seen ended shortly thereafter in April of 1865.

Mary's service during the war had not gone unnoticed, and both General Thomas and General Sherman nominated her for awards. After a review of her case, it was recommended by an official report to President Andrew Johnson that Mary should be officially recognized. Seven months later on November 11, 1865, President Johnson presented Mary with the highest award lauded for bravery, the Congressional Medal of Honor.[37]

The official citation reads, in part: "Whereas, it appears from Official Reports that Dr. Mary E. Walker, a graduate of medicine of the Medical School at Syracuse, New York, has tendered valuable service to the Government and her efforts have been earnest in a variety of ways and that she was assigned to duty and served as an Assistant Surgeon...in the service of the United States and has devoted herself with patriotic zeal to the relief of our sick and wounded soldiers, both in the field and hospital, to the detriment of her own health, and has also endured hardships as a prisoner of war....Whereas in the opinion of the president, an honorable recognition of her services and sufferings shall be made...and that the usual medal of honor for meritorious services be given to her." President Johnson and Edwin Stanton, Secretary of War signed the proclamation. [38] This was Mary's proudest moment, and one that the famous Civil War photographer Matthew Brady would capture for her. At that moment she became the first, and remains the only, woman to be so honored.

From this moment, Mary became a national celebrity overnight. She was soon recognized in major cities all along the east coast. She was a popular choice for headlines in local papers around the country, mostly for her idiosyncratic ways of life. There was nothing comparable to the sight of the indomitable spirit of Dr. Mary Walker.

The *Richmond Bulletin* reported the sight of "Miss Dr. Mary E. Walker" shortly after the end of the war in the summer of 1865. It was described as quite an attraction as Mary walked through the city's streets " ... clad in a blue coat with military buttons, and a very long skirt, a pair of nicely fitting blue pants...and gaiters, which fitted so as to display a pretty foot. As she passed ... her retinue in number would have done no discredit to a lieutenant-general. Ladies congregated upon the corners, and men and boys stopped along the sidewalk to comment upon the novel appearance of a lady in uniform." The procession was interrupted as "she turned to go through the market, she was stopped by the provost-guard, who asked her by what authority she appeared upon the streets in the garb in which she was attired. She replied, 'By what authority do you make the inquiry?' Guard — 'By order of the Provost-Marshal.' 'Then give him my compliments and tell him I will call upon him.' She then moved off as if nothing had occurred." [39]

Dress Reform & Suffrage

After the war, Mary resumed her efforts towards dress reform and the suffrage movement. Before and during the war, Mary had written articles for a progressive women's magazine titled *Sibyl*. One of her articles read in part: "Never until women are better educated physiologically, until they are considered something besides a drudge or a doll—until they have all of the social, educational and political advantages that men enjoy—in a word, equality with men, shall we consider vice in our sex more culpable than a man." [40] Mary urged women to "throw aside their embroidery, and read Mental Philosophy, Moral Science and Physiology, and then go to a smith's and have their dressical and dietitical chains severed that they may go forth free, sensible woman." [41]

She soon became a member of the National Dress Reform Association and at an 1860 meeting in Waterloo, New York, was elected as a vice-president. In 1866, she was called by a former *Sibyl* magazine associate, Dr. Lydia Hasbrouck, to "work in earnest upon the...woman's right to vote and the dress question." [42] She was eager to help and arrived in New York City in June of 1866.

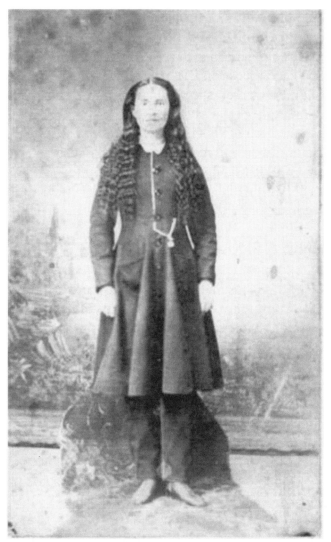

Figure 11: This photograph of Dr. Mary Walker was taken in Natchez, Mississippi during a lecture tour of the Midwest and Southern states in 1869-1870. This is a one-piece bloomer dress with a lace collar and pants beneath. Even though Mary wore the bloomer dress with pants, her long, wavy hair still provided a very feminine appearance. Courtesy of the Oswego County Historical Society Collections.

While shopping at a millinery store her "bizarre" costume began to interest several onlookers and soon created a crowd. "Dr. Mary was arrested ... for impersonating a man. She defended herself briskly, calling the female corset she abhorred a 'coffin contrived of iron bands.' The swaying, leg-revealing hoop skirt she termed as an invention of the 'prostitutes of Paris.'" [43]

Mary filed charged against the arresting officer and her case was brought to court. Needless to say, Mary defended her attire wholeheartedly. The commissioner of the case replied to Mary's defense of her dress by saying, "I consider, Madam, that you have as good a right to wear that clothing as I have to wear mine, and he [the defendant] has no more right to arrest you for it, than he has me. But if you were creating a disturbance ... he would be justified in removing you." The commissioner concluded by saying, "You are smarter than most ladies in the City of New York. I would have no hesitation in letting you go your own way ... but he [the police officer] thought you a weak woman needing protection. [To the policeman] Let her go, she can take care of herself. Never arrest her again." [44] She left the proceedings under applause of the crowd.

Mary was soon after elected president of the National Dress Reform Association. Later in 1866 at a dress reform convention in Syracuse, New York, the society congratulated the press of New York City "for the able manner in which they have defended Dr. Mary E. Walker for advocating the inherent right of women to dress in the manner that comports with freedom of motion, health and morality." [45]

Mary wrote adamantly about the subject of dress reform. "The greatest sorrows from which women suffer today are those physical, moral and mental ones, that are caused by their unhygienic manner of dressing! The want of the ballot is but a toy by comparison." [46] But Mary's radicalism would not stop here.

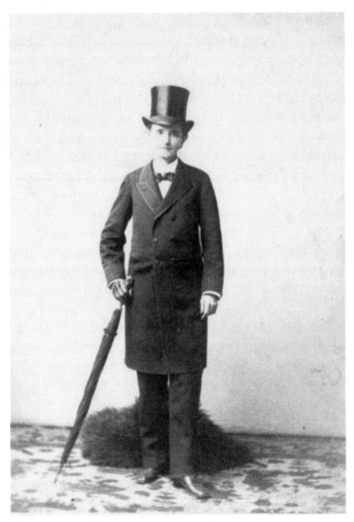

Figure 12: This is one of the earliest photographs taken of Dr. Mary Walker after her drastic turn to masculine attire. The long frock coat, pants, bow tie, top hat, gloves and umbrella date the picture to the early 1880s. Here Mary is in her forties and by this time has also changed her appearance further by cutting her long hair. It is this style of dress that found Mary the subject of gossip and ridicule. Courtesy of the Oswego County Historical Society Collections.

Eventually she abandoned the bloomer costume, popularized by some of the early suffrage leaders, including Elizabeth Cady Stanton. By the 1880s her attire was unquestionably masculine. By this time she donned a top hat, dress pants, vest, tailcoat and a bow tie. At this point, Mary had completely surpassed all boundaries of acceptable female fashion. In one incident "the Chinese Minister to the United States, Wu Ting-fang, asked Mary why she wore pants.

'Why do you wear a skirt?' she parried.

'It is the custom of my country,' the dignified Wu answered.

'It is the custom in my country to do as one pleases,' quipped the irrepressible Mary." [47]

There was a small group of people through the years that were supportive of Mary, even if they didn't always agree with her ideas and beliefs. Among this minority group was Mary S. Logan, a former Civil War nurse and wife of a Civil War General and U.S. Senator John Alexander Logan from Illinois. Mrs. Logan eventually became an author of women's history, wrote several books, and had this to say about Mary, "Because of her determination to wear male attire, Dr. Walker has been made the subject of abuse and ridicule by persons of narrow minds. The fact that she persists in wearing the attire in which she did a man's service in the army blinds the thoughtless to her great achievements and her right to justice from our government." [48]

In September of 1866, Mary was invited to England "to serve as a delegate to a social science congress in Manchester, England." [49] Her invitation soon turned into a nationwide tour of England. She soon became an English celebrity, lecturing on platforms to audiences who came to see this anomaly of an American female doctor. She then continued on to France before returning to the states. "She had arrived in England unheralded. By dint of her self-confidence and poise, durability and adaptability, her flair for the dramatic, and of course, with a big assist from her bizarre costume, she had taken old England by storm—a truly notable achievement," [50] Snyder wrote.

At home she was much less respected and was often the victim of vicious pranks. In July 1870, one of the many such incidents in her life was brought to action in the local police court in Oswego. While walking in downtown Oswego, a sixteen-year-old boy turned a water pipe on Mary as she passed him by. The boy claimed it was an accident, but Mary contended it was no mistake.

"The evidence of the Doctor and another witness was taken as to the circumstances the former contending that the act was intentional from the fact that the perpetrator of the trick observed its effect with a malicious smile," read one newspaper account. The defense counsel "animadverted upon the eccentricities of the complainant, and ventured to ask Doctor Walker if she considered that her style of attire was calculated to command public respect and consideration. The Doctor replied sharply that it was none of his contemptible business."

While Mary was not asking for severe punishment for the boy, she strongly expected "some expression that would indicate a due regard for the rights and privileges of society, and a determination to protect all of its members in their enjoyment." In short, she wanted to be respected and treated just like others, without fear of being attacked based on what she wore. She also stated "it was her pleasure to wear an American costume, adapted to her ideas of comfort, elegance and convenience ... "

She consistently and adamantly "demanded to be protected in that privilege, until such times as woman should assert and demonstrate her right to participate in framing and enforcing the laws under which she had to live." [51] The boy testified in his own defense and protested earnestly that the whole incident had been an accident. The court decided to give him the benefit of the doubt. This was yet another defeat for Mary.

In 1871, Mary would write her first book, entitled *HIT: Essays on Women's Rights*. As one biographer Susan Waters wrote, "Modern-day readers might be surprised to find that *HIT*, despite its nineteenth-century writing style, reflects many feminist ideas today." [52] Mary had much to say in her book on women's issues, especially suffrage. She was particularly clear that women were robbed of the right to vote, and there was only one thing in the way — men. Mary argued that it was only the men in political power who kept women from their right to vote. She stated, "That the Political equality of the sexes will produce radical changes in society generally and the marriage relation specially, is evident to all." [53] This she argued was the principle reason men did not want to give women suffrage; all because of the probability of a shift in power:

"Power always carries with it a certain amount of re-spect, whether it be of brain, body, purse, or Ballot...it matters not how much of all other powers one has, if deprived of the ballot..." She continued by addressing her opponents head on. "Men of America — you have robbed us of our most precious inheritance...That you are our protectors, is not true; for if you were, who would there be to protect us from?"[54]

Her strong views of tolerance and equality in relation to other subjects, also shines through in her writings. Other topics she covered in *HIT* with fervor included religion. "As there is something good in all religious beliefs, there should be a quiet tolerations towards all who represent the various forms of worship." [55] Mary expressed a nondenominational religious faith in her writings. "Now I am a member of every church in a sense. I have lived to see good in every church, and to see good in every kind of an association, and to affiliate with everything that is for the good and elevation of humanity." [56] She also believed that, "No Religion is true and genuine...unless it makes homes happy, and enables life generally...as embodied by the golden rule." [57]

After her eventful lecture tour in England, Mary returned to America to join the pioneers in the women's suffrage movement. She became actively involved in the Central Women's Suffrage Bureau in Washington, D.C. and appeared at Congressional hearings. She jointly advocated feminist causes with attorney Belva Lockwood. She also shared a home with Lockwood, who ran for president of the United States in 1884 and 1888. [58]

Mary was in the midst of the women's rights movement, making appearances with many of the well-known suffragists including Lucy Stone and Susan B. Anthony. She was receiving much attention and had been invited to receptions held by presidents and first ladies since Abraham and Mary Lincoln. In fact, Mary was invited and attended President Ulysses Grant's inaugural ball. [59] A report circulated in the *New York Times* in 1869 that stated, "Mr. Grant refused to meet Mrs. Dr. Walker unless she abdicated the terrors of her trousers and her umbrella, and come to him clothed in the usual garments of her sex." [60] Mary denied such reports and said that she had attended several receptions at the White House and had always been treated courteously.

In that same year, Mary participated in the Cincinnati suffrage convention along with Lucy Stone and Susan B. Anthony. She continued a speaking tour in 1870 promoting suffrage for women. Her adventures also made occasional appearances in the local media of Oswego, which often noted the whereabouts of their native daughter: "Dr. Mary Walker, having completed her Canadian tour, was registered at Bagg's hotel, Utica, yesterday, in company with Hon. Susan B. Anthony." [61]

Mary spread her message to women wherever she would be heard: "Struggle for political rights, for it is through such, and such alone, that you will ever obtain human rights.

It is not simply for yourself, but for that great army of young women who cannot yet see the necessity for anything but smiles and gallantry from their future husbands." [62]

Mary, along with Belva Lockwood, Frederick Douglass and many others, led a march in Washington in 1871 to claim their right to vote. The group presented a petition and asked to be registered. After the officials refused, Mary said, "Gentlemen, these women have assembled to exercise the right of citizens of a professed-to-be republican country, and if you debar them of the right to register, you but add new proof that this is a tyrannical government, sustained by force and not by justice. As long as you tax women and deprive them of the right of franchise, you but make yourselves tyrants. You imprison women for crimes you have forbidden women to legislate upon." [63] Needless to say, the march failed. In 1872, she unsuccessfully attempted to vote in Oswego, as did Susan B. Anthony in Rochester. [64]

She would repeat the attempt to vote more than once. In the November election of 1880, Mary appeared once again at the local polls in the town of Oswego. The inspectors once again denied her right to vote, stating that she was not legally qualified. A local newspaper covered the story:

"She insisted on her right to vote, and the oath respecting the qualification of the voter being read to her, she said: "I am a fe-male citizen and therefore a male citizen."" Mary's frustration would continue further when the other male voters noticed she failed in her attempt to vote. "Some pert young fellow in the crowd said if she was going to vote, they might as well dress all their women folks in men's clothes and bring them down and vote them. 'I don't wear men's clothes,' retorted Dr. Walker, sharply, 'I wear my own clothes.'" [65]

She continued to travel in the circle of other well-known suffragettes like Elizabeth Cady Stanton, Victoria Woodhull and others. At a Woman Suffrage Convention in

Washington, D.C., in 1872, Mary was a featured speaker. In fact, a fellow presenter speaking on spiritualism and sociology was "hissed and hooted of the stage amid repeated cries of 'Dr. Mary Walker — Dr. Walker!'" [66] Her colorful speaking style and unusual manner of dress made her a crowd favorite.

As time went on, the suffrage leaders eventually requested the government to pass a declaratory law, one that officially acknowledged the right to vote, regardless of race or sex. In 1877, as a member of the Women's Suffrage Association, Walker testified before the Judiciary Committee of the House of Representatives to support woman suffrage. She also prepared handbills, dispatched memorials to Congress, spoke at fairs and Grange halls, as well. "But the failure to obtain the ballot through mass registrations and the declaratory act convinced most of the suffragists that success hinged upon an amendment to the Constitution ...." [67]

However, Mary refused to follow this course of action. " ... She maintained till the end of her life that "We the people" included women, and therefore women already possessed the right to vote." [68] She argued: "I am opposed to granting men the right to vote on the rights of women. It is an unconstitutional usurpation of power." [69] The conservative leaders of the movement, including Lucy Stone and Susan B. Anthony, soon began to disassociate themselves with Mary.

Soon she was disassociated from the organization altogether. Her choice in apparel and her aggressive manner were among the reasons support for her ideas declined. However, the principal reason was that the suffrage leaders planned to achieve their goal through a constitutional amendment. Mary emphatically opposed any amendment proposals and would spend the remainder of her life fighting for her right to vote alone. "Typical of Mary's tenacious belief that the world could be changed was her prophecy that the time would come when men and women would be socially and politically equal and that 'men would be astonished that they could have opposed what was really for their own interest, as well as that of women'," wrote Waters. [70]

Many of Mary's prophecies did come true in time. Among the many topics she discussed in her book *HIT*, and preached in her lectures eventually became realities. Her beliefs on dress reform, that women should abandon corsets and petticoats became a reality with the gradual philosophical change in female fashion. Ironically, in modern times almost every woman owns a pair of pants. Yet, Mary endured constant ridicule for what she wore. Her writings also predicted the achievement of suffrage, although not in the way she wanted. The reality was granted with the passing of the 19th Amendment to the United States Constitution.

Mary also addressed temperance and the use of alcohol. She recognized a growing social issue that revolved around the abuses of alcohol. Mary especially focused on how it affected the family unit. "Think of how many families have suffered by deaths from Intemperance—how many marriages been severed!" [71] she wrote. "It is not necessary to use liquors of any kind to the extent that will produce entire, or even partial intoxication, to make a great amount of wretchedness, for the little that causes irritability, often makes more real and continuous unhappiness in the marriage relation..." [72]

Mary believed that the government needed to examine the issue of intemperance and get to the root of the problem, instead of building institutions for those affected. She wrote, "Government allows the poison to be made; and it licenses men to sell it to the people, and then it licenses Lawyers to defend those who commit crimes while under the effects of such poison, and it pays Policeman to watch them, and builds jails and prisons to confine the unruly...Government is altogether too dignified an institution, to look farther into the matter than to build poor-houses for the wives and children." [73] It would not be until the early 20th century when this issue eventually came to national attention and finally resulted in the 18th Amendment to the United States Constitution. With equal passion, she also preached on the evils of tobacco.

Even twenty years or more after she first appeared in trousers, Mary was still attracting public attention. She had many altercations due to her style of dress and was continually forced to fight for her right to wear pants in public. Her unusual appearance often caused much curiosity and drew large crowds that sometimes followed her around. In 1878, while simply walking through the streets of New York City, Mary again became a headliner in the *New York Times*.

A policeman stopped her and insisted that she tell him whether she was a man or a woman. She promptly told him to go along and mind his own business. After her remark, the policeman arrested her for disorderly conduct in being a woman wearing masculine attire. The officer took her to the nearest police station, but the officer in charge did not wish to take responsibility for adjudicating the case. Mary was then taken to police headquarters. There she met with the police superintendent, who told Mary that she had committed no offense and was free to go. Mary responded, "But this thing has got to stop. I'll carry a pistol and I'll use it if ever I'm interfered with again." [74] Over and over, Mary refused to give in.

By the 1880s, Mary's popularity as a public speaker for packed theater and lecture halls had subsided. The social issues she wanted addressed were no longer cutting edge and she had exhausted her audience. The leaders of the suffrage movement that had so often depended on her popularity and energy had long turned her away. She was still unwilling to accept the idea of an amendment to the United States Constitution that would allow women the right to vote. She stood by her belief that it was unnecessary, as she believed the Constitution already provided women the right to vote. Regardless of her opinions, the majority of the suffrage leaders had

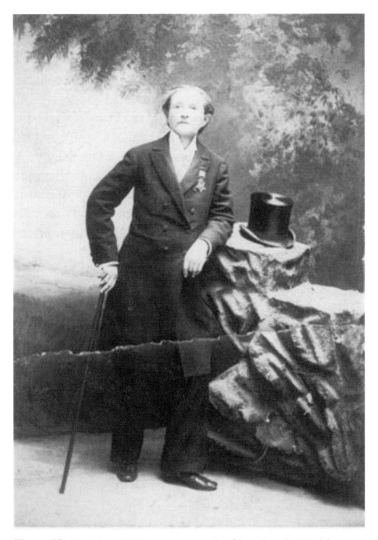

Figure 13: Dr. Mary Walker spent much of her time in Washington, D.C. visiting the U.S. Capitol when Congress was in session. This photograph taken in 1898 in Washington, D.C. shows Mary at about age 65. Beginning in the 1870s she began to dress in masculine attire and would continue to do so for the rest of her life. This was an expression of freedom in the style of dress. Mary almost always wore a top hat and carried an umbrella or walking stick, as displayed here. As in many of her photographs, she is also proudly wearing her Medal of Honor. Courtesy of the Oswego County Historical Society Collections.

long decided the way to achieve their goal was through a constitutional amendment.

In the 1880s, Mary first signed up to appear in a Dime Museum, a traveling sideshow with mixture of performances and lectures given to a middle class audience. It was far from the great lecture halls of Great Britian and France where she had achieved notoriety after the Civil War. She dismissed the idea that lecturing in a Dime Museum was a step backward on her part and stated, "I am of the opinion that the crying need of the masses is a better and more thorough scientific education than they at present receive ... I want to instruct a class of people who cannot afford to patronize high-priced lectures." [75]

While home for Mary was the family farm on Bunker Hill in Oswego, she spent much of her time in the nation's capital. She was typically seen during the times when Congress was in session and was a regular sight in the U.S. Capitol. Mary was the ultimate lobbyist of her day, always fighting for the issues she believed in. She was a solitary force and worked alone. She was commonly seen in political functions at the local, state and national level.

Frequent mentions of her were made in the local and national newspapers on her activities while in Washington. One report in 1899 read: "Dr. Mary Walker came into the Capitol today for the first time this session...She sent her card to several Senators, but they were all too busy to see her." [76] Sadly, this would be a habitual pattern in her later years. Most of the political leaders had already seen and heard her before and would not indulge her ideas.

The Later Years

Even though Mary's critics by far outnumbered her admirers, there were believers who no doubt fueled Mary's ambitions:

"One of these days," wrote one soldier Edwin DeFoe, "when some enterprising individual undertakes to write the history of this rebellion [you will] figure very conspicuously, as one who has done much good for the wives and widows of the soldiers ... " [77]

An article published in *The New York Times* in 1912 read: "Few people have ridiculed Dr. Mary to her face ... just why it would be hard to say. Perhaps it was because she had a sort of dignity, and because about her essential "goodness" there has never been any question." [78]

The story of Dr. Mary Walker is one full of exciting and sometimes amazing events. Yet there is a voice of sadness in its narration:

"Presidents and cabinet ministers and great generals were glad to meet and listen to me," Mary said. "I was younger then, and I was working for our soldier boys, just as so many girls and young women are working in the Red Cross for our boys who are over there [in Europe during World War I]. But now I am alone with the infirmities of age fast weighing me down and practically penniless, and no one wants to be bothered with me. But it is the same experience that has come to others, and why should I complain?" [79]

One final blow to Mary's pride, especially that of her service in the war, was the notice in 1917 that she was among 910 Medal of Honor recipients to have their award revoked. This determination was based on a review board's report that Mary had been a civilian contract surgeon, not an enlisted soldier; and also that there was insufficient evidence supporting the honor. The committee requested the return of her original 1865 medal and another medal that had been issued in 1907 with a new design. She refused to return either of the medals and declared, "One of them I will wear everyday, and the other I will wear on occasion." [80] They were never taken from her.

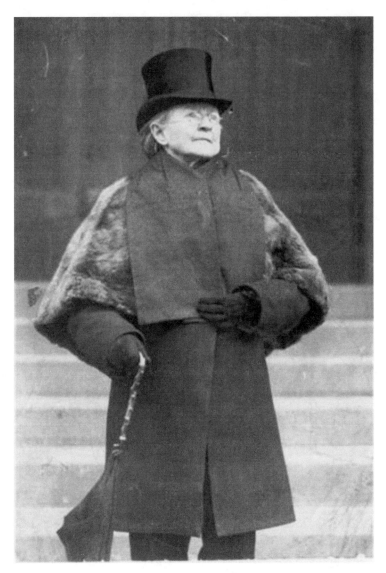

Figure 14: Dr. Mary Walker is shown here in this undated photograph taken later in her life, circa 1910, with her signature top hat, largely out of use in everyday male attire by this time. The fur cape and scarf indicate that the photograph was taken during the colder months, possibly in Oswego. Although Mary went through an evolution of styles and taste in fashion, her masculine form of dress is the one she is most remembered for. Courtesy of the Oswego County Historical Society Collections.

Two years later Mary died on February 21, 1919, at the age of 86. Her death came just one year before the ratification of the 19th amendment, giving American women the right to vote. In this way, her life is full of irony. She never lived to see her "golden hopes with dreams secure," [81] as she once wrote. Yet, she seemed always instinctually sure that her ambitions for women would be realized, even if it were after her lifetime. She was buried with her parents in the Oswego Rural Cemetery in a black frock suit. [82]

Examining the life of such a unique person gives a stronger perspective of history. In retrospect it is hard for a modern reader to understand the trials and tribulations Mary faced. The rights she desired and fought for until death are mostly taken for granted in the 21st century. It is because of this that she is often remembered for her peculiarities instead of her wisdom, her masculine attire instead of her personal style, and her eccentric behavior instead of her passion for the American dream. Often the echoes of her dissenters still carry over so long after her death. However, she is equally remembered as a woman who was courageous, strong and undying in her devotion.

In an interview in her later years, Mary said these prophetic words: "I have got to die before people will know who I am and what I have done. It is a shame that people who lead reforms in this world are not appreciated until after they are dead; then the world pays its tributes by piling rocks over the grave of the reformer. I would be thankful if people would treat me decently now instead of erecting great piles of stone over me after I am dead. But, then, that's human nature."[83]

Remembering Mary

After her death, decency and the basic rights she so desired would come true. Even though the 1917 Medal of Honor review board revoked her honor, the next generation would carry on her battle to have the award reinstated. After a long process, Mary's grandniece Helen Hay Wilson was able to provide substantial documentation showing a wrongful termination of her award. In 1977, the Army Board of Corrections of Military Records finally reinstated Mary's status on the Medal of Honor rolls. [84] Remarkably, out of the approximate 3,200 Medal of Honor recipients to date, Dr. Mary E. Walker is the first and only women recognized in American history.

In 1962, Charles McCool Snyder wrote the definitive biography on Mary's life entitled *Dr. Mary E. Walker: Little Lady in Pants*. Snyder pieced together her life from beginning to end through countless resources and separated the myth from the woman. In 1964, the Dr. Mary Walker Health Center at the State University College at Oswego was built and dedicated in her honor. The center serves as a clinical health facility for students at the university in memory of Mary. A New York State Historical Marker was placed at the site of her birthplace and family farm on Bunker Hill.

In 1982, Walker was honored with a commemorative stamp by the United States Post Office in recognition of her life and accomplishments. The stamp was released on the 150th anniversary of her birth. In 1990, a play entitled "Champion Bold: Dr. Mary Walker Speaks" was written and performed by Rosemarie Imhoff and Mark Cole in Tyler Hall at Oswego State University. More recently her life was featured in Elizabeth Leonard's 1994 book entitled *Yankee Women: Gender Battles in the Civil War.* The book chronicles the lives of three women, including Mary, who provided their services for Union forces in the Civil War.

After several nomination attempts, Mary was finally inducted in the year 2000 into the National Women's Hall of Fame in Seneca Falls, NY. In 2001, historian Mercedes Graf wrote *A Woman of Honor.* The book chronicles Mary's military years, including most of Mary's own personal memoirs of her Civil War experiences. In the same year, a mural of Mary by artist Ellen Klem was unveiled in downtown Oswego as part of the Oswego Mural Project commissioned by the Greater Oswego Chamber of Commerce.

In 2002, Chapter One of the book *Medal of Honor* by Allen Mikelian featured her story as the only woman in American history to receive the Medal of Honor. She is also remembered through the Dr. Mary E. Walker Award, which recognizes and rewards outstanding army spouses and civilians with the U.S. Army Military District of Washington, whose volunteer achievements merit special recognition. Mary's book *HIT,* originally released in 1871, was republished in 2003. Another biography of her life by historian Dale L. Walker titled *Mary Edwards Walker: Above and Beyond* was released in 2005. In these ways, her story continues with countless tributes after her death.

An admirer, only known as Mr. Herron, once wrote these words to Mary, "...for sometime yet you will be the target, as you have been heretofore, for unreasonable criticisms, slanders and falsehoods. But I feel confident that your convictions as to what is right and sensible will sustain you in still pursuing a straight-forward, independent course. The self- sacrifices you have made will yet receive their proper acknowledgment and you will live when your maligners are dead and forgotten." [85]

Bibliography

Filler, Louis. *Notable American Women 1607-1950*. New York, 1971.

Groat, Charles. *Dr. Mary Walker: A Reader*. Oswego, 1994.

Leonard, Elizabeth D. *Yankee Women*. New York, 1994.

Mikaelian, Allen. *Medal of Honor: Profiles of America's Military Heroes from the Civil War to the Present*. New York, 2002.

Snyder, Charles M. *Dr. Mary Walker: Little Lady in Pants*. New York, 1962.

Walker, Mary E., M.D. *Hit*. New York, 1871.

Waters, Susan C. "The Invincible Doctor Walker." *New York Alive* (Nov./Dec. 1983): 30-33.

Wright, Fred P. "Dr. Mary E. Walker." *Bicentennial Journal of the Oswego County Historical Society (1976-1977):* 146-155.

Notes

1. Mary E. Walker, M.D., *HIT, Essays on Women's Rights* (1871; reprint, Amherst, NY: Humanity Books, 2003), 34.

2. Walker, 115-116.

3. Charles M. Snyder, *Dr. Mary Walker: Little Lady in Pants* (New York: Vantage Press, 1962), 13.

4. *The Minneapolis Tribune,* July 4, 1897 (Oswego County Historical Society Collection).

5. Elizabeth D. Leonard, *Yankee Women: Gender Battles in the Civil War* (New York: W.W. Norton & Company, 1994), 106.

6. Snyder, 14.

7. Ibid., 16.

8. Leonard, 109.

9. Snyder, 17.

10. Ibid., 17.

11. Ibid., 18.

12. *The Oswego Palladium,* December 7, 1855, p. 2 (Justin D. White Collection).

13. Snyder, 18.

14. Leonard, 111.

15. Walker, 43, 51.

16. Ibid., 45.

17. Ibid., 142.

18. Ibid., 142.

19. Ibid., 80.

20. Leonard, 249.

21. Ibid., 112.

22. Ibid., 121.

23. Mercedes Graf, *A Woman of Honor: Dr. Mary E. Walker* (Gettysburg: Thomas Publications, 2001), 36-37.

24. Ibid.

25. Ibid.

26. Leonard, 119.

27. Ibid., 131.

28 Ibid., 132.

29. Graf, 53.

30. Leonard, 135.

31. Ibid.

32. Snyder, 41.

33. Leonard, 139.

34. Snyder, 35.

35. Mikaelian, Allen. *Medal of Honor: Profiles of America's Military Heroes from the Civil War to the Present.* New York, 2002.

36. Leonard, 141.

37. Mikaelain, 12.

38. Official Citation, original in collection of Oswego County Historical Society.

39. *The New York Times,* July 9, 1865, p. 8 (Justin D. White Collection).

40. Snyder, 23-24.

41. Ibid., 24.

42. Ibid., 56.

43. Groat, Charles. *Dr. Mary Walker: A Reader.* Oswego, 1994: 24.

44. Snyder, 59.

45. Ibid., 60.

46. Walker, 80.

47. Snyder, 139.

48. Leonard, 105.

49. Snyder, 61.

50. Ibid., 77.

51. *The Oswego Daily Advertiser & Times,* July 1, 1870, p. 3 (Justin D. White Collection).

52. Waters, Susan C. "The Invincible Doctor Walker." *New York Alive* (Nov./Dec. 1983): 30-33.

53. Walker, 119.

54. Ibid., 134.

55. Ibid., 167.

56. Source Unknown.

57. Walker, 170.

58. Louis Filler, *Notable American Women 1607-1950* (New York, 1971), p. 532.

59. Snyder, 88-89.

60. *The Oswego Advertiser & Times,* April 7, 1869, p. 4 (Justin D. White Collection).

61. *The Oswego Advertiser & Times,* Dec. 22, 1870, p. 4 (Justin D. White Collection).

62. Waters, 30.

63. Snyder, 95.

64. Ibid., 97.

65. *The Oswego Daily Palladium,* November 4, 1880, p. 4 (Justin D. White Collection).

66. *The New York Times*, January 13, 1872, p. 4 (Justin D. White Collection).

67. Snyder, 98.

68. Ibid., 100-101.

69. Snyder, 103.

70. Waters, 32.

71. Walker, 108.

72. Ibid., 109.

73. Ibid., 112-113.

74. *The New York Times,* December 6, 1878 p. 2 (Justin D. White Collection).

75. *The New York Times,* March 8, 1887, p. 1 (Justin D. White Collection).

76. *The Oswego Daily Palladium,* January 19, 1899, p. 4. (Justin D. White Collection)

77. Leonard, 126.

78. Ibid., 105.

79. Snyder, 151.

80. Ibid., 54.

81. Fred P. Wright, "Dr. Mary E. Walker," *Bicentennial Journal of the Oswego County Historical Society (1976-1977):* 146-155.

82. Graf, 88.

83. *The Minneapolis Tribune,* July 4, 1897 (Oswego County Historical Society Collection).

84. *The Washington Post,* Saturday, June 11, 1977, p. A3.

85. Waters, 33.

All the Heaven I Want

The Life of Dr. Sarah Loguen Fraser

by Susan Keeter

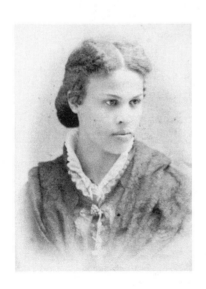

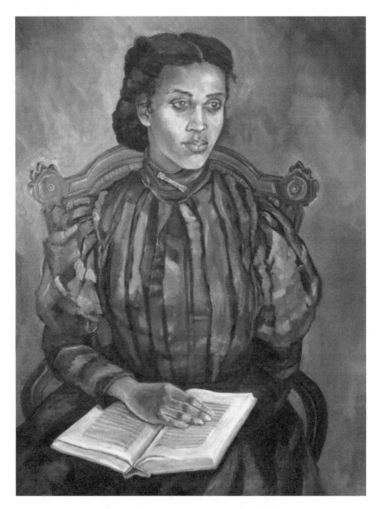

Figure 15: Sarah Loguen Fraser, MD, class of 1876. Oil paint on canvas by Susan Keeter, 2000. Courtesy Syracuse Medical Alumni Association/SUNY Upstate Medical University.

Previous page: Sarah Loguen, early 1880s. Courtesy Goins Papers, Moorland-Spingarn Research Center, Howard University.

"From the first day *I saw you...I have dreamed of tow-headed pink-faced youngsters, you the mother, I the father...a man picks a wife and mother to his children not on account of race, but because something higher dictates...marry me,"* implored Edward Stone, a respected white physician, when he encountered Sarah Loguen in Syracuse's Fayette Park in summer 1876.

Dr. Stone's request for marriage had been proceeded by the insistence that Dr. Loguen give up her plans to practice medicine, with the rationale that "women doctors are considered curiosities, freaks, unsexed creatures."

According to her family papers at Howard University, Dr. Loguen responded, "My home and family have been a beacon to light the way for the poor, oppressed, and hunted of (my) race. The time has passed for the need of shelter, but God knows, we need to build strong and healthy bodies. To have those of my race come to me for aid — and for me to be able to give it — will be all the Heaven I want."

"You'll have a damned hard time in your heaven," huffed Dr. Stone.

To the average 21st-century school girl, it seems

89

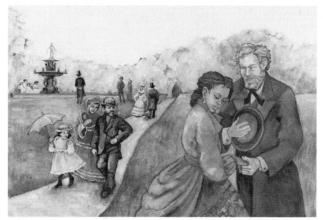

Figure 16: Sarah Loguen and Dr. Stone, Fayette Park, Syracuse, New York. Oil paint on paper by Susan Keeter, 2004.

obvious that Dr. Loguen would reject Stone's offer in favor of an internship at a Philadelphia hospital. But, consider his proposal based on the limitations and expectations of 19th century America. The Civil War and slavery had ended, but women could not vote or own property. Her parents were dead, and her older sister had married and moved away. She was a 26-year-old, unmarried African American woman at a time when only ten percent of Americans had a high school education and the life expectancy for African Americans was 33 years.

Dr. Loguen's refusal was a reflection of her life-long commitment to social justice and personal achievement.

Sarah Loguen was born in 1850, the year the Fugitive Slave Act was enacted, and was the daughter of the Reverend and Mrs. Jermain Wesley Loguen, leading abolitionists in Syracuse who helped 1,500 people escape slavery. She witnessed the Civil War; the devastation caused by cholera, scarlet fever and tuberculosis; the benefits of Reconstruction; the invention of the telephone, typewriter, and electric light; the

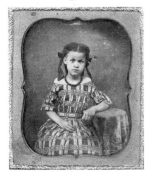

Figure 17: Sarah Loguen, 1857. Courtesy Goins Papers, Moorland-Spingarn Research Center, Howard University.

discovery of the role of germs and the development of pasteurization; World War I; and the Great Depression.

She was raised and educated in Syracuse, New York and became one of the nation's first African American women doctors. At 32, she moved to Santo Domingo, now the Dominican Republic, and became the first woman physician in that country. At 44, she became a widowed pharmacy- and plantation-owner, as well as a doctor. And, long after she could have retired and lived comfortably on her accumulated wealth, Dr. Loguen Fraser volunteered as a doctor at a Women's Clinic in Washington, D.C. She died in 1933, the year Franklin Delano Roosevelt was elected president.

The Reverend's Daughter

Sarah Loguen was born literally in the midst of one of the most passionate times of conflict between slavery and abolition. According to her unpublished 1933 biography, *Underground Railroad Princess*, a large meeting was held at the Loguen home the evening before she was born. Its purpose was to organize the fight against the impending Fugitive Slave Act, a law that strengthened the ability of slave owners to go into free states to regain their "property." There were jail sentences and huge financial penalties for people who harbored escaped slaves. Sarah's family was particularly vulnerable, both because their home was Syracuse's main station of the underground railroad and because her father, the Reverend Jermain Wesley Loguen, was a fugitive slave.

Sarah was a toddler when her father was a leader in the "Jerry Rescue" (October 1851), a defiant act that freed an imprisoned former slave, garnered national attention, and forever weakened the fugitive slave law. Arrest warrants were issued for those involved, and Sarah's mother convinced Reverend Loguen to leave home for the safety of Canada. One evening, an armed crowd gathered in front of the Loguen house, fueled by a false rumor that Reverend Loguen had been arrested while trying to return from Canada. Mrs. Loguen and the children waited anxiously for word of Reverend Loguen, who quickly returned home to comfort his family. Once there, he picked up little Sarah, who was feverish with measles, and "so frightened and trembled so violently, that he held her in his arms for the best part of the night."

While Reverend Loguen was safe that time, the threat of penalites and imprisonment remained. Sarah's mother,

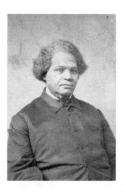 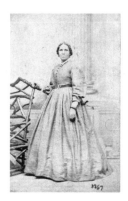

Figure 18 (left): Sarah's father: The Rev. Jermain Wesley Loguen. Courtesy Goins Papers, Moorland-Spingarn Research Center, Howard University.
Figure 19 (right): Sarah's mother: Caroline Storum Loguen. Courtesy Goins Papers, Moorland-Spingarn Research Center, Howard University.

Caroline Storum, decided to talk with the Loguen children about slavery and the danger of working against it. Her mother counseled, "Should any strangers question (you), talk freely about (me and our) family, but be silent about (your) father —where he is, how he is, what he is doing. Notice how many and where the strangers were, what they looked like, then run home and tell (me) right away."

The Underground Railroad caused a great polarization among people. There were many, like Secretary of State Daniel Webster, who saw protecting the rights of slave owners as the duty of law-abiding citizens. And there were others, like Gerrit Smith, who gave their fortunes to abolitionist causes and risked their safety by participating in illegal actions to help people escape slavery.

Throughout these volatile times, Reverend Loguen flaunted his opposition to slavery by giving powerful public speeches asserting that "God had made (all men) free" and that he would not dignify the cruelty and injustice of slavery by allowing his freedom to be purchased. He used the pulpit to taunt law enforcement and slave owners with (to paraphrase), "You want to capture a slave? Here I am!"

Raised in the UGRR Depot

When Sarah Loguen was six, her family's underground railroad work —although it remained illegal —was conducted quite publicly, as evidenced by the following excerpts from 1856 Syracuse newspapers:

> *Chronicle*, Jan. 22:
> We had the pleasure of seeing seven...fugitives fresh from the land of the "Peculiar Institution,"...(They) arrived at Loguen's last night, where they were cared for, and are probably now on their way to the Land of the Free. Two of them were married to-day.

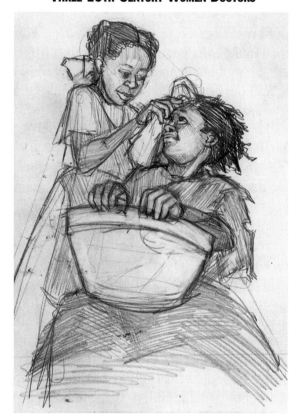

Figure 20: Young Sarah Loguen caring for child who had escaped slavery. Sketch by Susan Keeter, 2001.

Journal, April 11:
Two brave fellows arrived at the Underground Depot last night...Our friend Loguen, the agent for this line, in this city, took them in charge and saw them well provided for. One of these fugitives started from his 'master's' premises with a pair of handcuffs on...he was relieved of (them in Philadelphia)...and declared a freeman.

Standard, May 31:
The tide of travel on the Underground Railroad is increasing. Eight colored passengers went through this

city yesterday, on their way to Canada....Liberty operates like a magnet....and draws (one)...to the land where they don't sell babies at auction.

Journal, July 18:
So great has been the colored migration from the land of chains lately that J.W. Loguen has been obliged to visit Canada and provide a house, where the(y)... may go...until they are prepared to seek employment....This indefatigable agent (Mr. Loguen) deserves great credit on behalf of his outraged countrymen....

Standard, Aug. 23:
We saw Brother Loguen in the Depot yesterday with $4,800 of Southern Currency. It consisted of four able bodied men, and one young woman, valued at home at the above sum....

Through her parents' anti-slavery work, Sarah Loguen was acquainted with a number of influential people including Frederick Douglass, Gerrit Smith, Harriet Tubman, and John Brown. She was nine when John Brown led the raid on Harper's Ferry (in October 1859). Immediately after the raid, tensions were high and the government was looking for accomplices. To protect her father, Sarah Loguen helped burn all her father's correspondence with John Brown. Reverend Loguen and several other abolitionist leaders fled to Canada.

Several weeks later (on December 2, 1859), John Brown was executed and Syracuse mourned. Businesses and churches were draped in black, flags were hung at half-mast, and church bells tolled. A memorial service was held, which Sarah attended with her family.

Sarah Loguen's father was emboldened to write the following, which was published in Frederick Douglass' abolitionist newspaper, *The North Star*. "We thank God that...such a man as John Brown lived....Virginia may think she has put him to death, yet he lives...in the hearts of every liberty-loving individual in our country."

By age ten, Sarah had learned that following one's beliefs could put one squarely in conflict with societal norms. Her parents' work on the underground railroad taught Sarah that, not only was it God's will and every person's duty to help others, but it was her responsibility to accept sacrifice and face opposition.

Family Matters

Sarah's mother, Caroline Storum Loguen, was the daughter of abolitionists from western New York. She made the Loguen home a meeting place for antislavery and religious groups and refuge for 1,500 fugitive slaves. She was a friend of a group of Iroquois women who shared herbs and herbal medicine remedies which she used to treat the injuries and illnesses of fugitive slaves.

In addition to her own eight children, Sarah's mother raised Henry Kelso, a teenaged fugitive slave; Josephine Storum, a distant niece; and Julia Luckett, the 'sickly' daughter of a friend. Since the Reverend Loguen travelled frequently, much of the care of the fugitives must have fallen to Sarah's mother. There were meals to cook; donations of clothes to be collected, washed, and sewn; illnesses and wounds to be treated; farm animals to raise; vegetable gardens to tend; and travel arrangements to be made.

A graduate of Oneida Institute, Sarah's mother was a wise and dignified woman. As a symbol of the importance the Loguens placed on the people they were helping, she recorded the names of all the visiting fugitives with a gold pen in the leather-bound 'hotel registry.' Mrs. Loguen tutored her children and instructed them on the importance of "pure thoughts and good penmanship."

Sarah was the fifth of the eight children of Jermain and Caroline Loguen: Elizabeth Letitia (b. 1841), Helen Amelia (b. 1843), Gabriella Clorinda (b. 1845), Gerrit Smith (b. 1847), Sarah Marinda (b. 1850), Jermain William (b. 1851), Mary Catherine (b. 1853) and Cora Juliette (b. 1859). Gabriella died at age 2, several years before Sarah was born.

Sarah Loguen never met her paternal grandmother, Jane McCoy, but learned about bravery and the crippling effects of servitude through stories of her grandmother's life. Jane McCoy, whose slave name was Cherry, had been born free in Ohio around 1791 but was kidnapped and sold into slavery when she was seven years old. Ten years later, Cherry was impregnated by her master's teenaged son, David Logue, who fathered Reverend Loguen, as well as his younger brother and sisters. There are accounts of Sarah's grandmother threatening and beating the plantation overseer when he tried to harm one of her children. Cherry's fierce protection of them ended when she was beaten almost to death fighting, unsuccessfully, to prevent slave traders from taking two of her children to sell at auction. When Sarah was a child, Reverend Loguen made attempts to free his mother from slavery. Her masters, the Logue family, knew of Reverend Loguen's firm belief that freedom was a God-given birth right, not a privilege to be purchased. They made Grandmother Cherry's freedom impossible by 'agreeing' to release her, but only on the condition that Reverend Loguen return to the slave state of Tennessee to buy the privilege of his freedom.

Sarah Loguen's maternal great-grandmother, Mary Ann (Polly) Fowler, was a white French Canadian woman who, in the late 1700s, raised four sons with her free African/ Native American common-law husband, Charles Storum. She travelled by oxcart, and was described as vivacious, with curly black hair and silk stockings. During Sarah's childhood, her 'taciturn Aunt Tin' admonished Sarah for any display of self-confidence or original thinking with, "It's the Polly Fowler in you that makes you have such silly notions."

Sarah responded, in thought only, "I'm glad Polly had the gumption to do what she pleased and live her own life."

Aunt Jule, Caroline Loguen's younger sister, Juliette Clorinda Storum, visited the Loguens frequently, helped care for fugitive slaves, and shared her love of nature with Sarah. They went horseback riding together and Aunt Jule taught Sarah to recognize bird songs, identify trees, and appreciate the scents of apples and other fruit. This early education may have helped Sarah Loguen later as she studied botany in medical school.

When Sarah Loguen was ten, her father—who had been living free for 25 years—received a letter from the wife of his former master, Mannasseth Logue. "In consequence of you running away," Mrs. Logue wrote, "we had to sell Abe and Ann (his brother and sister) and 12 acres of land." She admonished him by writing that, as a preacher, he should read his Bible and to repent by sending her $1,000 so that she could buy back the 12 acres of land. If not, she would be forced to get the $1,000 by selling Reverend Loguen to another slave master.

In response, Reverend Loguen wrote, "I stand among a free people, who, I thank God, sympathize with my rights and the rights of mankind...if you...come to re-enslave me, and escape the unshrinking vigor of my own right arm, I trust my strong and brave friends will be my rescuers and avengers."

The Value of Education

Sarah Loguen was able to break barriers and attend medical school, in part, because she came from a well-educated family. Her father understood the liberating power of education. He had been raised as an illiterate slave but was introduced to the alphabet— and philosophical debate—in his late teens by a Methodist family who had leased him from his master. This exposure to education, and some civility, prepared Sarah's father to escape slavery. Once living in freedom in Hamilton, New York, Sarah's father learned to read and write. He became a college student at the Oneida Institute in Whitesboro and it was there that he met Sarah's mother, Caroline Storum.

Sarah Loguen's early education was strong. She began attending schools in Syracuse at age five and was tutored by her family when they had extended visits at her materal grandparents' home. As teenagers, the Loguen children's education included Shakespeare, French, chemistry, and trigonometry. She also studied German, the language in which the most advanced and influential medical texts were written.

As part of their commitment to helping others, the Loguens established schools in Syracuse for African Americans. *The Syracuse Journal* (April 7, 1864) described the Loguens' role in education:

"Sufficient credit is not generally given to the colored people for their efforts to obtain an education...(A)t the evening schools a goodly number of adults make considerable sacrifice for the sake of improving...These evening schools are mainly in the charge of Miss Loguen (21-year-old sister, Amelia), daughter of Rev. J.W. Loguen...the organization of these free schools is due more to the efforts of Mr. Loguen than to those of any other person..."

Witnessing War

It was the first year of the Civil War and 11-year-old Sarah Loguen was playing outside with a friend. They heard moaning and discovered George Clark, a Union soldier, nearly drowned, hiding in their well. He was a teenaged neighbor who had fled from his regiment after his first experience with the trauma of battle. Sarah and her friend tried to help George themselves, but Sarah's mother came to the rescue, pulled the mud-covered George out of the well, and helped him to his mother's back door. Knowing that a soldier's penalty for desertion was likely death, Mrs. Loguen told the girls, "You have seen no one. Say nothing about this to anyone, understand? "

George's mother, Melly Clark, was a close friend of Sarah's mother and supporter of the Loguens' antislavery work. She nursed her son back to health and encouraged him to go back to fight in the war. Not long after, he was declared missing in action and Mrs. Clark turned to Caroline Loguen — and Sarah — for solace. For years, Mrs. Clark searched for her son among returning soldiers, but he was never found.

The Loguen family received news from the Civil War battlefield from sergeant-major Lewis Douglass, sister Amelia's fiancé and son of Frederick Douglass. From Morris Island, South Carolina (on July 20), Douglass wrote a letter describing two battles in which 300 men had been killed, and included a list of friends who were missing or wounded. The letter closed with, "Remember if I die, I die in a good cause. I wish we had a hundred thousand colored troops. We would put an end to this war."

In 1864, when Sarah Loguen was 14, the Civil War was at its height and Syracuse was so "unsettled and unsafe" that Sarah, her mother, brothers and sisters went to live in Busti (in western New York, near Jamestown) with her maternal grandparents.

The Civil War ended a year later. Union soldiers including friends and neighbors, were returning home— wounded, missing limbs, mentally ill. There was an outbreak of cholera in Syracuse. The sick were quarantined and swamps were drained in an effort to contain the disease. Three months after Sarah turned 15, and less than a week after the end of the Civil War (April 14, 1865), President Abraham Lincoln was assassinated in Washington, D.C. Sarah Loguen may have paid her respects as Lincoln's funeral train wove its way through Syracuse.

Illness and Loss

It is likely that Sarah Loguen chose medicine as her path for helping others because she had witnessed suffering and faced terrible personal losses at the hands of disease. She was five when her older sister, Letitia, died of heart failure. Imagine that sad child shuttled off to an aunt's house while her 13-year-old sister lay in a casket in the parlor of her home, surrounded by geraniums and pine boughs, with a stream of visitors offering sympathy to her parents.

Ten years later, Sarah Loguen's mother, Caroline, was stricken by tuberculosis, a rampant disease for which there was no cure. Weakened and bedridden, she relied on Sarah to care for her and run the household. When Caroline Loguen died in 1867, her body was laid out on the couch in the back parlor, as had been done when Letitia died. Several of Mrs. Loguen's friends kept all-night vigils and for days, Sarah's father locked himself in the upstairs bedroom.

With her mother gone and her older sister, Amelia, planning to marry and move away, Sarah was left with running the Loguen household and assisting with her father's ministry. A year after her mother's death, Sarah graduated from high school and Reverend Loguen accepted the appointment as bishop of the African Methodist Episcopal Zion church.

Bishop Loguen's ministry required that he travel extensively. There is a poignant moment in *Underground Railroad Princess* in which Sarah Loguen begged to join her father on an upcoming trip. He declined, insisting that he would return soon. Sarah accompanied him to the train station and tearfully bid him farewell. A few days later, she received news that her father has been stricken with a heart attack in Saratoga, New York, and died. Sarah was 22.

Pivotal Moment

According to the *Underground Railroad Princess*, a single incident pushed Sarah Loguen to become a doctor. In spring 1873, she was at a crowded railroad station in Washington, D.C. when she noticed a young boy running between carriages and wagons, earning money by offering grain to horses. Sarah was collecting her luggage and chatting with friends when she heard screams, the screech of wagon wheels, and the squeal of horses being reined in. The child had been run over and pinned under a farm wagon. Others heard the child's screams and gathered to gawk at the accident. Sarah searched for a doctor but could find none. Eventually, the station master was found, and the injured child was carried away, screaming.

Once on her train, Sarah sat with eyes closed, absorbing the terrible event, and remembering her mother's words, "Nothing that is human do I reckon is beyond my concern."

Sarah Loguen vowed, "I will never see a human being in need and not be able to help" and concluded that, "We turn to God with spiritual trouble and to doctors with physical trouble."

She would become a doctor.

A Mentor Found

At some point during the trip, her family physician, Dr. Michael Dunning Benedict, boarded the train. He sat with Sarah Loguen and questioned the seriousness of her pledge by asking, "Have you any idea what being a doctor means?"

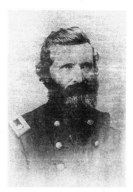

Figure 21: Major Michael D. Benedict, M.D., 75th NYS Volunteer Infantry Regiment. Courtesy U.S. Army Military History Institute.

Dr. Benedict had been an underground railroad agent in Skaneateles, New York and a surgeon in the 75th Infantry during the Civil War. His valet during the war had been Henry Kelso, a young fugitive slave raised by the Loguen family. Dr. Benedict was an agent of the Freedmen's Relief Society which helped "colored" people find employment after the war. In 1867/8, Benedict had tried, unsuccessfully, to get a woman doctor accepted into the Onondaga County Medical Society. As a member, he had pushed for the medical society to accept the credentials of women's medical colleges and made statements for the record that qualifed women were being excluded from mainstream medicine solely because of gender. He was a respected physician in Syracuse and on the faculty of Syracuse University's College of Medicine.

After a long discussion, Dr. Benedict agreed to tutor Sarah Loguen in preparation for medical school. For the next five months, she devoted herself to study, meditation, exercise, and a vegetarian diet.

At that time, doctors were battling many diseases, few of which were actually treatable. (The discovery of penicillin was more than 50 years in the future.) The medical community, however, was quarantining sick people to reduce the spread of infectious disease and working to change the water supply to stop outbreaks of cholera, malaria, and typhoid fe-

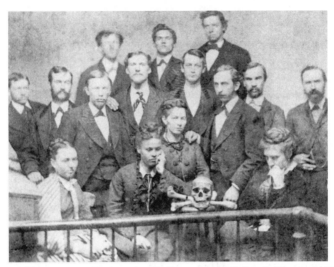

Figure 22: Syracuse University College of Medicine,* Class of 1876. Sarah Loguen, center front. (*now SUNY Upstate Medical University College of Medicine) Courtesy Goins Papers, Moorland-Spingarn Research Center, Howard University.

ver. A vaccine for smallpox had been invented, and it was given to school children. Sadly, tuberculosis, typhus, measles, whooping cough, diphtheria, and scarlet fever were rampant, and 75 percent of children died before the age of five (Benedict talk, 1873).

Medical School

> " We understand that Miss Sarah M. Loguen, daughter of the late Bishop J.W. Loguen, has commenced the study of medicine under the tuition (sic) of Dr. M.D. Benedict of this city. This is woman's rights in the right direction and we cordially wish this estimable young lady every success in the pursuit of the profession of her choice."
>
> —*Syracuse* (New York) *Journal*, October 1873 (the

year that Sarah Loguen became one of the first African American women in the United States to attend medical school)

When Sarah Loguen began medical school, the college of medicine at Syracuse University had been open for a year. It had been purchased from Geneva College by Syracuse University, and the new location offered clinical experiences at St. Joseph's Hospital, which had opened in 1869, and the House of the Good Shepherd and City Hospital, both of which opened while Sarah was a student. The medical school at Syracuse, in keeping with those at Harvard University and the University of Chicago, offered the most rigorous program of study available at the time: three years of study, with examinations, to earn a medical diploma.

There were 18 doctors on the faculty and 17 students in Sarah Loguen's first-year class, including four women. The first day began at 8 a.m. with a lecture by Dr. Benedict and a tour of the medical school building which consisted of class-

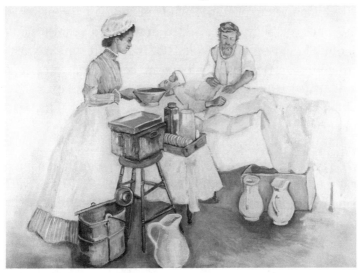

Figure 23: Medical student Sarah Loguen assisting Dr. Michael Benedict in surgery. Oil paint on paper by Susan Keeter.

rooms, a lecture hall, dissecting room, and an operating room. First-year courses included anatomy, physiology, histology, chemistry, and botany. The faculty and students wore long white aprons to dissect cadavers in the anatomy class and, for comfort, the women students did not wear bustles under their dresses.

During the second year of medical school, Sarah and her classmates had more coursework in anatomy, chemistry, and *materia medica*. They began assisting in surgery. Anesthesia consisted of an ether- or chloroform-soaked rag stuffed in a metal funnel and held near the patient's nose and mouth.

The medical students also accompanied their professors on afternoon hospital visits. The House of the Good Shepherd (now University Hospital) provided medical care to 'charity' cases. At City Hospital, commonly known as the pest house, they cared for people suffering from infectious diseases like scarlet and typhoid fevers, malaria, diphtheria, and small pox, which had reached epidemic proportion.

Courses in obstetrics and gynecology, forensic medicine, and psychiatry were added in the third year of medical school. Sarah Loguen attended her first birth, which was performed by Dr. Benedict, and among her clinical experiences were visits to the Syracuse insane asylum. Final exams were held in January 1876 and students were notified of the results in February.

At a small ceremony in a faculty office, Dr. Benedict asked each graduating student to, "Raise your right hand, repeat the Hippocratic Oath," and said, "By the power vested in me by the Trustees of the Medical School of Syracuse University, I confer on you, the degree of Doctor of Medicine."

At the end of the office ceremony, Dr. Benedict shook each student's hand, then asked Sarah Loguen to stay behind. Privately, he said to her, "I am proud of you, as I know your father, Bishop Loguen, would have been. May God bless you."

That small ceremony was followed by a graduation at

the Weiting Opera House in Syracuse. Considered one of the finest in the country, it was adorned with stained glass lamps and crystal chandeliers, monogrammed staircases, velvet and gilt, and handpainted back drops on the stage. Huge vases of flowers decorated the theater and an orchestra played music. Graduates wore black gowns and mortar boards and marched single file to receive their diplomas from Chancellor Erastus Otis Haven. When Sarah Loguen was handed her doctor of medicine diploma, the audience broke into applause. According to the *Underground Railroad Princess*, "They had not forgotten Bishop Loguen, and that was his daughter."

Sarah Loguen sent graduation announcements to many people, including Frederick Douglass' son, Charles, who worked at the American Consulate in Santo Domingo and was a friend of pharmacist Charles Fraser.

After graduation, Dr. Benedict encouraged Sarah Loguen to apply for internships at the New England Hospital for Women and Children in Boston and the Women's Hospital in Philadelphia. Without her knowledge, Dr. Benedict sent a letter of recommendation to the Philadelphia hospital and went there in person to discuss her qualifications with the staff. Sarah was offered the internship.

'Miss Doc' in Philadelphia

Dr. Sarah Loguen arrived at the Women's Hospital of Philadelphia in September, accompanied by Mrs. Fuller, a family friend who had been active in the abolitionist movement when Sarah was a child. They arrived at the three-story brick building carrying Sarah's trunk, which was filled with medical books, a doctor's kit, copy of the Hippocratic Oath, sewing box, family photos, book of Longfellow's poetry, and a prayer book.

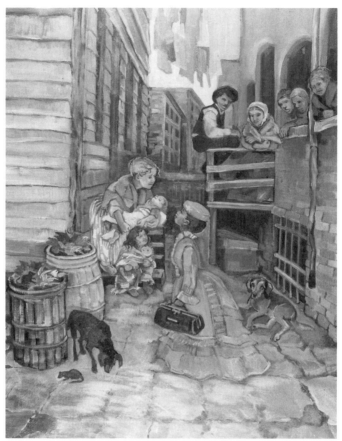

Figure 24: Dr. Sarah Loguen ("Miss Doc") does house calls in Philadelphia's Commons, 1876-1877. Oil paint on paper by Susan Keeter.

Dr. Loguen's introduction to this hospital internship was less than welcoming. She was to work with an intern named Dr. Logue, who left the hospital 'because' of Sarah. As soon as she arrived, the hospital staff noticed the resemblance in appearance and names between Sarah Loguen and Dr. Logue, a young white intern from Nashville, Tennessee. Sarah knew that her own father was born in Manscoe Creek, a few miles from Nashville. It became obvious that the two doctors were related through David Logue, Sarah's father's

slave master and biological father. The white Dr. Logue —
distressed by evidence that she shared a heritage with this
'colored girl' — took ill, shut herself up in her room for days,
and left the internship.

Dr. Sarah Loguen and the remaining interns lived in
small furnished rooms on the third floor of the hospital and
ate their meals in the basement. The operating room and patient rooms were on the second floor and consultation rooms,
an office and pharmacy were on the first.

On the first day of work, Dr. Hester Greenly took Dr.
Sarah Loguen on a tour of the hospital and to the Commons,
a neighborhood served by the hospital and described in the
Underground Railroad Princess as full of "hovels of Irish
squatters, stagnant water, patches of weeds, pig pens, dogs
and dirty children." On that day, Drs. Greenly and Loguen
were greeted by a mass of children, eagerly shouting, "Hello,
Miss Doc, Hello, Miss Doc," "Mom's got a fever," "Tim's a
nail in his foot," and "Mom says come fix Pop's and her's
heads." They spent a long day, moving from one family to
another, cleaning wounds and dispensing medicine and sympathy.

The following day, the internship began in earnest.
Dr. Sarah Loguen received a long list of duties from the medical director with the message, "May your courage and ardor
never be dimmed."

One afternoon in November, Sarah returned from a
long night and full day of caring for sick people in the Commons to find a calling card from a Mr. Charles Fraser of Santo
Domingo, who had waited three hours to visit with her. He
was travelling in the U.S. and had also visited her brother,
Gerrit, and sister, Mary Catherine, at the suggestion of their
mutal friend, Charles, son of Frederick Douglass.

On Valentine's Day, 1877, Sarah wrote a letter to her
sister, Amelia. In it, she described church services, encoun-
ters with friends, efforts to decorate her meager living quar-

ters, and her life as a hospital intern.

> Dear Sister - Meal: (Amelia)
> ...We are having terrible times here now. Three of the assistants out of four have given up sick. ...Two of us have the work of five. ... when you are going all day and are called up and out two and three times in the night one is apt to feel tired. ... I had my second pair of twins Sunday night....I have to manage to make ends meet and I do not succeed always. Once in a while I can get a patient to pay me car fare, then I walk and have the money...I try to get along but it is hard pulling. ...The dinner bell is ringing and I am almost as hungry as I can be....Sometimes I cannot stand it and I go and buy three cents worth of crackers and eat them on the street. I should faint - but for it ....
> Give my love to all....
> Affectionately, Tin (her family's nickname for Sarah)

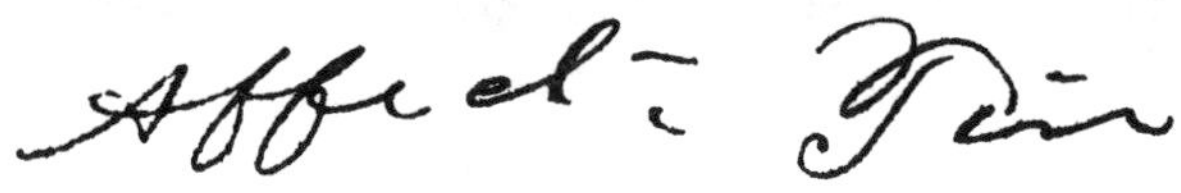

Figure 25: Detail of Letter. Courtesy Goins Papers, Moorland-Spingarn Research Center, Howard University.

That year, Rutherford Hayes became president and recently attained civil rights for African Americans were being dismantled. It was the beginning of the end of an era described by Hedda Garza (in *Women in Medicine*) as, "...the atmosphere immediately after the Union victory left a tiny crack in the wall through which a handful of black women slipped."

During this time, Sarah Loguen and Charles Fraser

began to exchange letters, photographs and gifts. Frederick Douglass, in a fatherly and pointed manner, let Sarah know that he liked Fraser's home, Santo Domingo (Dominican Republic), because "There you feel your full stature of manhood."

New England Intern

In fall 1878, Dr. Sarah Loguen moved to Boston to fill a six-month vacancy at the New England Hospital for Women and Children. There was no salary, but comfortable living quarters, sufficient food, and a more supportive environment there. The hospital was founded in 1862 by Dr. Marie Zakrzewska, a former colleague of Elizabeth Blackwell's, in an effort to raise academic standards and increase opportunities for women in medicine. The year Sarah arrived in Boston, the first women's medical society in the U.S. (the New England Hospital Medical Society) was established there, with Dr. Zakrzewska as president. The New England Hospital had an all female staff and after 1881, only women with medical degrees were accepted. The first professional nursing school in the country began at the New England Hospital and it accepted the first African American nursing students.

D.C. Doctor

Dr. Sarah Loguen moved to Washington, D.C. during the summer of 1879. Several years earlier, the National Medical Society had been established in the District of Columbia for African American physicians—male and female—because they were excluded from the American Medical Association.

Dr. Loguen opened her first doctor's office in the front

room of a private home in Washington, D.C. and Frederick Douglass installed her office sign, saying, "There is your shingle, now for your work."

Dr. Loguen built her practice by assisting a Dr. Parson on her cases. Gradually, Sarah became family physician to many prominent Washington families and had men, women, and children as private patients, but she was allowed to treat only women and children in hospitals. Her medical equipment would have consisted of racks of medicine bottles, a stethoscope, thermometer, tourniquets, syringe and needles, catheters, bandages, and adhesive. She would have carried a black bag to house calls, sterilized equipment on kitchen stoves, and performed minor surgery in patients' homes.

Exhaustion

After a couple of years, long work hours and exposure to disease and unsanitary conditions took its toll. Dr. Loguen contracted malaria and, in spring 1881, she went to Harper's Ferry to recuperate. She wrote Charles Fraser in Santo Domingo and let him know that she was ill and resting from overwork. He promptly wrote back and asked her to marry him. Along with the marriage proposal (in June 1881), he sent a newspaper article describing his new pharmacy building and noting that "The acquaintances of Mr. Fraser will be pleased to learn of...his material prosperity."

Friends and family were visiting when Dr. Sarah Loguen received the letter, and she showed it to Frederick Douglass who responded, "I advise you to answer favorably."

But, Charley Mitchell, Douglass' young nephew, complained, "If you go to Puerto Plata, I'm sure I'll never see you again for it must be further than heaven. I have heard of Heaven, but I never heard of Puerto Plata, Santo Domingo."

And Sarah's older sister, Amelia Loguen Douglass,

disparaged the marriage proposal by saying, "You better stop doing the spectacular" and "There's such a thing as taking the pitcher to the well once too often."

But Amelia's father-in-law, Frederick Douglass, answered firmly, "I have been to that part of the world and I know Mr. Fraser. If (Sarah) were my daughter, I would gladly consent to her marriage."

Dr. Loguen replied to Fraser's letter, but the slow transport of intercontinental mail and her hesitant response delayed the actual engagement for six months. Once Fraser understood that she had said "yes," he sent Sarah a heart-shaped emerald engagement ring with the message, "Green is love everlasting."

Dr. Loguen returned to her medical practice in Washington until the summer of 1882, when she went to Syracuse to help her younger sister, Mary Catherine, who was pregnant with her second child, and to prepare to marry in the fall.

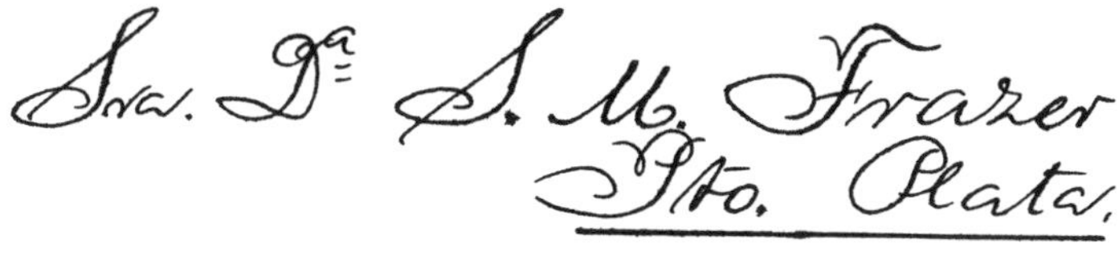

Figure 26: Detail of a letter. Courtesy Goins Papers, Moorland-Spingarn Research Center, Howard University.

A Husband and a Caribbean Home

Marriage to Charles Fraser offered the 33-year-old Dr. Loguen financial security, social standing, and professional prominence in a new culture. And unlike Dr. Stone, who had proposed marriage several years earlier, Charles Fraser believed in her as a doctor.

Charles Alexander Fraser was a pharmacist and plantation owner, friend of politicians and philathropists, and "a gentleman of pleasing countenance and keen intellect." Born in the West Indies, he was the eldest of three children. Their parents, Charles of Denmark and Dorothy of the Danish West Indies (now known as St. Johns), died during a smallpox epidemic. Fraser traveled extensively and donated West Indian artifacts to the Smithsonian Institute and Philadelphia's Institute of Natural History. He attended the Moravian church (German Protestant) and befriended Loguen family friend, Charles Douglass, by persuading him to join a group of men who built a church by literally hauling stones while singing hymns.

Sarah Loguen and Charles Fraser married on a stormy Tuesday in September 1882 in Syracuse, but according to the *Underground Railroad Princess*, "the wind and rain stopped and the sun shown through the church window on the bride and groom as they were pronounced man and wife."

The newlywed Frasers left that night for New York City. Charles Fraser wrote in his journal on the day of their marriage, "So at last I am married. God bless me and my wife," and on the following Sunday, "First Sabbath of my wedded life. May it be an inspiring day to my wife and me."

A New World

After a week in New York City, Charles and Sarah Fraser set sail for Santo Domingo. It was six days before they saw land, and Sarah's first glimpse of a Caribbean island. Their steamship moored and tiny rowboats flying English flags transported the passengers to the island so they could stretch and enjoy the palm trees, pink flamingos, and flowering cactus. Soon, it was back on the ship and two more days of travel to get to the country of Santo Domingo, and the Frasers' home on the northern coastal city of Puerto Plata.

When the Frasers arrived in Puerto Plata, a group of businessmen and government officials met them at the wharf to welcome them home and meet the bride. Dr. Sarah Loguen Fraser—in a black and white silk dress and matching parasol, lace gloves, and a hat adorned with fresh flowers and velvet ribbons—held her husband's arm as he made the formal introduction of "Gentlemen, Madame Fraser."

After going through customs, the Frasers walked the three blocks of main street to their home, where they were greeted by children tossing rose petals. The house and apothecary were filled with bouquets of flowers and neighbors brought cakes, more flowers, and tropical birds as welcome gifts. Charles Fraser owned Anacaona, a banana plantation and country home, as well as this red-tile-roofed city home and business.

Puerto Plata, the "Port of Silver," was the largest and most prosperous area of Santo Domingo. It was home to palm trees, rocky beaches, an extinct volcano, and fertile farm land. The wharf was used to export sugar, coffee, cocoa, and mahogany. The port city was a contrast of thatched roof huts and lavish white buildings with elaborate porches and wrought iron gates. People rode horses and oxen on the street and a train ran through the city. Spanish was the primary language, but French and English were spoken there as well.

The country of Santa Domingo had been a Spanish colony, and most residents were descendents of slaves. The indigenous people had been wiped out during Columbus' era. When Dr. Sarah Loguen Fraser arrived, the country was led by a dictator, Ulises Heureaux, who "although he did not achieve good government, he did provide enough internal order to encourage economic development." During his rule, a few short railways, telegraph and cable lines were completed and port facilities were improved, but the country's foreign debt increased tenfold.

Moving to the Caribbean was an adventure and an adjustment for Dr. Sarah Loguen Fraser. Her new neighbors thought it odd that she walked in the rain with an umbrella. She had to learn to manage house servants and watch for tarantulas hiding under water gourds and wash stands.

Dr. Loguen Fraser had a daily Spanish-language tutor. Since she had studied German and French as a teenager, Sarah quickly learned to read and write in Spanish. But, the spoken language was difficult for her, particularly because men's and women's inflections were different. Fortunately, a little neighbor girl befriended Sarah and patiently taught her to speak and hear Spanish.

Santo Domingo's First Woman Doctor

In April 1883, seven months after arriving in Puerto Plata, Dr. Loguen Fraser traveled to the capital, Santo Domingo City, to take an examination so that she could practice medicine in her new home. She brought her diploma and medical records, as well as the tortoise-shell handled medical tools that were a gift from her husband.

Her examination was held at the University of Santo Domingo, considered "the first center of learning in the new world." It was a grand place: a block-long Greek-style temple with a jade fountain in the center and Moorish adornments throughout. She was questioned at length, in Spanish, by the rector in charge of the university and eleven other men. Sarah left her patient histories for further examination and waited for the next steam ship to take her home.

It was six months before Dr. Loguen Fraser received the document, bearing the Domincan coat of arms, which authorized her to treat female patients and male and female children. The Dominican newspapers announced that Dr. Loguen Fraser would begin practicing medicine and she was

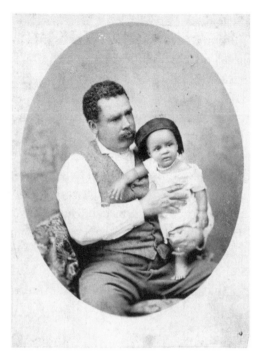

Figure 27: Charles Fraser and Gregoria Alejandria Fraser, Dr. Sarah Loguen Fraser's husband and daughter. Gregoria was the author of her mother's unpublished biography, *Underground Railroad Princess*. Courtesy Goins Papers, Moorland-Spingarn Research Center, Howard University.

immediately flooded with patients. Until she arrived, the only physicians in Puerto Plata were a French male doctor and a government doctor.

She was pleased to resume working as a doctor, but during that time, she learned that her younger brother, Will, had died in Syracuse.

Baby Gregoria

That December (1883), the Frasers' only child, Gregoria Alejandria, was born. She was a healthy and beautiful baby and Charles showered Sarah with gifts of diamond jewelry.

But the birth had been very difficult, and was assisted only by a country midwife because no doctor was available. Sarah was left unable to bear more children.

Frederick Douglass was Gregoria's godfather. The little girl's first language was Spanish. Her father spoke to her in Danish and her mother in English when she was very young. When Gregoria turned four, the Frasers decided to speak only English at home.

In fall 1884, the Frasers moved to a new house. Sarah planted fruit trees and flowers and decorated the yard with caged parrots, mockingbirds, and canaries. This new home was built with a doctor's office for her, which included separate examination and treatment rooms. Sarah saw patients there and was able to do house calls because Charles bought her a horse so that she could travel to see patients in the countryside.

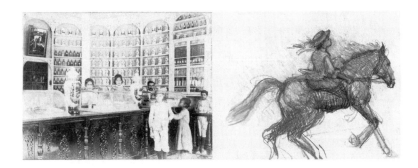

Figure 28 (left): Charles Fraser's Pharmacy, Puerto Plata, Santo Domingo. Courtesy Goins Papers, Moorland-Spingarn Research Center, Howard University.

Figure 29 (right): Dr. Sarah Loguen Fraser travels on horseback to make house calls to patients in the Dominican countryside. Sketch by Susan Keeter.

On one such trip, at the written request of General Bonilla, Dr. Loguen Fraser traveled 15 miles on horseback to care for his baby goddaughter. She arrived at the thatched-roof cottage to the sound of people wailing. The little girl had died before Sarah could help her.

Practicing medicine had its heartaches, but Dr. Loguen Fraser continued to work as a doctor, at the same time devoting herself to raising their daughter, being a good wife, assisting in the pharmacy, and managing their homes.

In 1885, there was more sad news from the Loguen family. Sarah's youngest sister, Cora Juliette, had died at age 26, shortly after giving birth to her only child, Leon Loguen Foster.

Discoveries and Set Backs

The 1890s were a time of tremendous advances in medicine. Pasteur had discovered that bacteria caused infection, Morton was developing anesthesia, Semmelweis was battling childhood fever, and Lister was promoting antisepsis in surgery. The medical profession finally understood that germs spread disease. People began to live longer.

At the same time in the United States, the majority of

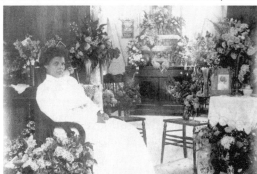

Figure 30: Sarah Loguen Fraser, Puerto Plata, Santo Domingo. Courtesy Goins Papers, Moorland-Spingarn Research Center, Howard University.

Reconstruction-era civil rights laws had been repealed and racial segregation had become a legalized reality in the south.

And, Sarah's family had more grief to bear. In September 1894, her 54-year-old husband, Charles, died of a stroke. Sarah, Gregoria, their minister, and several friends were at his bedside when he died. Sarah held her 11-year-old daughter (called Doe for her large brown eyes) and lamented, "Doe, I have to be in the Botica (drugstore) to take your father's place. You will take my place here. Mr. Dutton will tutor you daily from 10 to 12....I am so sorry..."

A year after her husband's death, Dr. Sarah Loguen Fraser sold the plantation, Anacaona. Two years later, she sold the pharmacy, as well, and rented their home in Puerto Plata. Sarah and Gregoria left Santo Domingo and traveled.

By 1899, the *Syracuse Journal* described Dr. Sarah Loguen Fraser as "a woman of considerable wealth" and a "member of a famous colored family." She and her daughter Gregoria were living in Washington, D.C. Gregoria was a student at Howard University and Sarah was living with her older sister, Amelia, and her husband, Lewis Douglass. Sarah still owned the Fraser family home in Santo Domingo but the country was in near anarchy. The dictator, Ulisses Heureaux, had been assassinated and there was no clear head of the country.

Sarah decided to move back to Syracuse, New York in 1901. She spent that Christmas with her brother, Gerrit; sister, Mary Catherine; and their families. It was their first holiday together since Sarah had married and moved to Santo Domingo almost 20 years earlier. Aunt Tin lived with her in the Westcott Street house, as did Gregoria, who was attending music school at Syracuse University.

For the next few years, Dr. Sarah Loguen Fraser moved between Syracuse, Washington, D.C., and Puerto Plata, caring for relatives and attending to her properties. In 1902, Henry Kelso, a horse trainer and former slave who had been

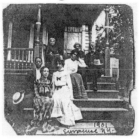

Figure 31: Dr. Sarah Loguen Fraser, with daughter and friends, Syracuse, New York, 1901. Courtesy Goins Papers, Moorland-Spingarn Research Center, Howard University.

raised by the Loguen family, returned to Syracuse to live with Gerrit Loguen's family. It was the first time that Sarah had seen Kelso in many years. Sadly, that same year, Gerrit's wife, Louise, died. By 1903, Sarah was back in Washington caring for her brother-in-law, Lewis Douglass, who had had a stroke. Sarah's daughter, Gregoria, had developed some mental health problems and the two traveled to Puerto Plata for a few months in 1904.

The following year, Heureaux's assassin, Ramon Caceres, assumed leadership of Santo Domingo. He reformed the constitution, set up a public works program, and led the country until he, too, was assassinated six years later. That September, Sarah's nephew, Gerrie (Gerrit's son), died of a pulmonary condition on a stretcher outside an Albany hospital. The hospital would not admit him because he was 'colored.'

Two years later (1907), Sarah Loguen Fraser was back in Syracuse, caring for her ailing younger sister, Mate (Mary Catherine) who died in March. Sarah sold the house in Syracuse and returned to Washington, D.C. to live with her sister, Amelia, and help care for Lewis Douglass, who had suffered a second stroke.

After Lewis died in 1908, Dr. Sarah Loguen Fraser, now in her late 50s, accepted a position as resident physician at the Blue Plains Industrial School for Boys. Her nephew,

Leon, and daughter, Gregoria, visited and were shocked to find that Dr. Loguen Fraser was expected to wash, iron, cook, and clean for 14 boys. Her daughter located the school superintendent and pronounced, "She was appointed resident physician, not cottage matron. Here is her resignation."

The superintendent responded, "She is appointed by the U.S. Government. The only way she can leave is to die."

"Consider her dead," answered Gregoria. They packed her mother's belongings and left.

Undeterred, Dr. Sarah Loguen Fraser continued to concentrate on doing good work and caring for her family. She was treasurer of the Order of the Malachites, a D.C.-based organization of African American accountants, lawyers and physicians. She volunteered two full days a week at a women's health clinic.

Sarah's older brother, Gerrit, now widowed and ill, moved to Washington to live with her. In 1917, her daughter, Gregoria, married John Goins. Sarah's brother, Gerrit, died a year later.

At age 69, Dr. Sarah Loguen Fraser still had a passport to travel to Santo Domingo to look after her property. In 1926, on the 50th anniversary of her graduation from medical school, the 76-year-old Dr. Loguen Fraser was the guest of honor at a Howard University alumni dinner. She wore a grey and pink silk crepe gown with lace.

Sarah lived the rest of her life in Washington, D.C. with her daughter, Gregoria, and her son-in-law, until John's death in 1930.

At noon on Palm Sunday (April 9, 1933), 83-year-old Dr. Sarah Loguen Fraser died at home with her daughter, Gregoria, holding her hand and light streaming in the window. Later, Gregoria wrote, "Thank God she went out in the sunshine."

Epilogue

Dr. Sarah Loguen Fraser was buried in Lincoln Cemetery in Washington, D.C., with a quiet graveside service attended by her daughter and few friends.

Meanwhile, in Puerto Plata, Dominican Republic, the Catholic Church held a high Mass and flags were hung at half-mast for nine days to mourn her death. Wreaths and flowers were placed on her husband's grave in remembrance of Dr. Loguen Fraser, the country's first woman doctor.

In Syracuse, New York, the newspaper published her obituary, although it had been decades since she had lived there.

> "Dr. S.L. Fraser Dead, Aged 83
> Woman Physician, Daughter of Negro Bishop
> She was born in this city January 29, 1850, and was graduated from the College of Medicine, Syracuse University, in 1876, one of the first women to be graduated from that college and one of the first Negro women in America to become physicians (sic). ...In 1882, she was married to Charles A. Fraser of Puerto Plata, a wealthy Negro, who died years ago...."

On her 150th birthday in 2000, Dr. Sarah Loguen Fraser was honored by her alma mater, now known as SUNY Upstate Medical University in Syracuse, New York. The celebration included a street renaming, the establishment of an annual named scholarship, a portrait dedication, installation of a historical marker, a lecture series, and a celebration attended by government officials and the medical community. Several magazine and news articles have been published on Dr. Loguen Fraser, and in 2003, an annual Sarah Loguen Fraser Day was established by medical students at SUNY Upstate.

And, Dr. Sarah Loguen Fraser has become the subject of elementary school history projects.

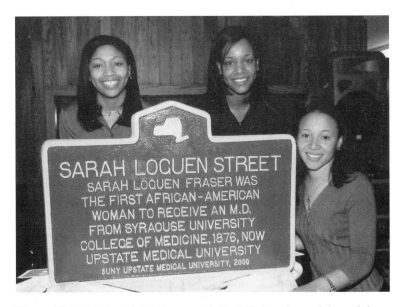

Figure 32: In 2000, SUNY Upstate Medical University celebrated the 150th birthday of Sarah Loguen, MD, class of 1876. SUNY Upstate Medical University students Renika McLeod, Tamika Oxford and Marcia Humphrey are pictured with the historical marker which was installed as part of her birthday celebration. Courtesy SUNY Upstate Medical University.

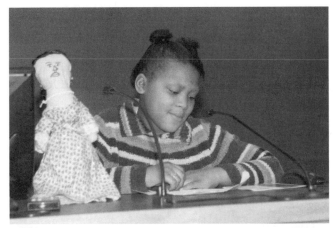

Figure 33: Shonquaysha Pate, a fifth grader from Dr. King Elementary School, read her essay on Dr. Loguen Fraser and showed the Dr. Loguen Fraser doll she created as part of a 2006 Dunbar Center history project. Courtesy SUNY Upstate Medical University.

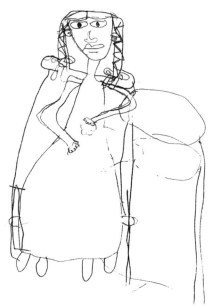

Figure 34: Sara Tucker was a second grader at Ed Smith Elementary School in Syracuse, when she created this drawing as part of her women's history project on Dr. Sarah Loguen Fraser. Courtesy SUNY Upstate Medical University.

Sarah Loguen Fraser Bibliography

BOOKS

Abrams, Ruth J. ed. *Send Us a Lady Physician: Women Doctors in America, 1835-1920*. New York: WW. Norton and Co., Inc., 1985.

Cohen, Daniel, *A History of Medicine*.

Garza, Hedd. *Women in Medicine*. New York: Franklin Watts, 1994.

Goins, Gregoria Fraser. *Underground Railroad Princess: Sarah Loguen Fraser, M.D.* Goins Papers, Moorland-Spingarn Research Center, Howard University, Washington, D.C. unpublished.

Hannau, Hans W. *The Islands of the Caribbean*. New York: Hastings House.

Haverstock, Nathan A. *Dominican Republic in Pictures*. Minneapolis: Lerner Publications, 1988.

Howard, Davis. *Dominican Republic: A Guide to the People, Politics and Culture*. New York: Interlink Books, 1999.

Hunter, Carol. *To Set the Captives Free: Reverend Jermain Wesley Loguen and the Struggle for Freedom in Central New York, 1835-1872*. New York and London: Garland Publishing, 1993.

Leslie, Edmund Norman. *History of Skaneateles*. New York: Andrew Kellog Press, 1902.

Loguen, Jermain Wesley. *The Rev. J.W. Loguen as a Slave and as a Freeman*. Syracuse: J.G.K. Truair, 1859/reprinted: New York: Negro Universities Press, 1968.

Luft, Eric v.d. *SUNY Upstate Medical University: A Pictorial History*. Syracuse: Gegensatz Press, 2005.

Metter, Zak. *Reconstruction: America After the Civil War*. New York: Lodestar/Dutton.

Petit, Eber M. *Sketches in the History of the Underground Railroad*. Westerfield, New York: Chatauqua Region Press, 1999.

Smith, H.P. *Syracuse and Its Surroundings: A Victorian Photo Tour of New York's Salt City*. Syracuse, New York: H. Child, 1878/ Reprinted: Syracuse,

New York: Black Dome Press, 2002.

Still, William. *The Underground Railroad*. Philadelphia: Porter and Coats, 1851.

Stringer, Helen Dann. *Millie, M.D., 1846-1927: The Story of a Nineteenth-Century Woman*. Utica: North Country Books, 1992.

Terkel, Susan Neiburg. *Colonial American Medicine*. Venture Books.

Wright, Kenneth W. *Foundations Well and Truly Laid: The Early History of SUNY Health Science Center at Syracuse*. Syracuse, Syracuse Medical Alumni Association, 1994.

Zeinert, Karen. *Those Courageous Women of the Civil War*.

ARTICLES

_____. Biotechnology Time Line. *The Post-Standard*, Syracuse, New York, Sept. 29, 2002.

_____. Welcome to the antiseptic nation. *The Post-Standard*, Syracuse, New York, January 19, 2004.

Luft, Eric v.d. Milestones in Pediatrics in Central New York. *Syracuse Medical Alumni Journal*, Spring 2004.

Luft, Eric.v.d. Sarah Loguen Fraser, M.D., Class of 1876: the College of Medicine's First African American Woman Physician. *Syracuse Medical Alumni Journal*, Summer 1998.

Palmer, Darlene. An Emphasis on Hygiene and Dreaded diseases. Elizabeth Blackwell: First Woman Doctor. *Cobblestone*, 2002.

Riede, Paul. Jerry Rescue sent a message to the nation, *Post-Standard*, Syracuse, New York, Oct. 29, 2001.

St. Marie, Satenig. The Family Doctor. *Victorian Home*. August 2004.

Wellman, Judith and Sernett, Milton. *Uncovering the Freedom Trail in Syracuse and Onondaga County*. Preservation Association of Central New York, 2002

Documents and Collections

Barnes Collection, Benedict Papers, History of Syracuse Hospitals, Loguen Family, Weiting Opera House, 19th C. Census Data, 1874 and 1910-1915 Census, Onondaga Historical Association Collection, Syracuse, New York.

Carter Godwin Woodson Collection of Negro Papers and Related Documents Library of Congress, Washington, D.C.

Fenton History Center Library, Jamestown, New York.

Gerrit Smith Papers, Special Collections Library, Syracuse Univerity.

Goins Papers, Moorland-Spingarn Research Center, Howard University, Washington, D.C.

Loguen Papers, Onondaga Historical Association Collection, Syracuse, New York.

Mary Burnham Family Papers, Private Collection of Nellie Burnham.

Michael D. Benedict Papers, Skaneateles Historical Society.

Mitchell, Mrs. O.W.H. Reminiscences of the University Hospital of the Good Shepherd, Syracuse University Alumni Program, December 2, 1966.

Oakwood-Morningside Cemetary Burial Records, Syracuse, New York.

Records of the Onondaga Medical Society, vol. II, 1851-1873 and vol. III, 1873-1878.

Special Collections, Health Sciences Library, SUNY Upstate Medical University, Syracuse, New York.

Storum Family Geneology, Private Collection of Jane Beecher.

INTERNET SOURCES

_____. Anesthesia.
www.people.virginia.edu/~wwc2r/vicstudies/anesthesia.html

_____. A Brief History of Crouse Hosptial.
www.crouse.org/aboutus/history.html

_____. The Common School.www.pbs.org/kcet/publicschool

_____. Dominican Republic. www.cia.gov/publications

_____. Freedom Trail. www.pacny.net/freedom_trail.loguen.htm

_____. From Quakery to Bacteriology: The Emergence of Modern Medicine in
19th Century America. University of Toledo Libraries.
www.cl.utoledo.edu/canaday/quakery

_____. Medicine of Jacksonian America. www.connerpraire.org/jmed.html

_____. New York History Net. www.nyhistory.com

_____. A Short History of Hospitals in Syracuse.
www.upstate.edu/library/history/hospitals.html

Cazalet, Sylain. New England Female Medical College and New England
Hospital for Women and Children. www.homeoint.org

Crowell, Kathy. The Medical Profession.
www.rootsweb.com/~nyononda/medicalprofession.html

Goodfellow, Sue. History of the Town of Skaneateles.
www.rootsweb.com/~nyononda/skaneat/ beauhit.html

Woodson, Carter. Beginning History of the African Methodist Episcopal Zion
Church, The History of the Negro Church. www.varickmemorialamezion.org

INTERVIEWS

Battle, Elizabeth.Town of Skaneateles Historian, ND.

Beecher, Jane. Storum Family History, ND.

Bodgan, Jane. Nineteenth-Century Childbirth in America, ND.

Burnham, Nellie. Mary Burnham and the History of Good Shepherd Home and Hospital, April 2004.

Luft, Eric v.d. Medical School, circa 1876, ND.

TALKS

Kay, Gwen E., Women in Medicine in the 19th Century in Onondaga County. Women in Medicine Professional Development Day, SUNY Upstate Medical University, March 13, 2006.

About the Authors . . .

Mary K. LeClair lives in Waterloo, NY, and works as an editor at Hobart and William Smith Colleges in Geneva, NY. She is a former newspaper journalist who enjoys discovering and researching women and men who have overcome remarkable obstacles in order to succeed. Elizabeth Blackwell, the first woman in America to become a physician, is one of these individuals. In 1849, Blackwell graduated from Geneva Medical College, the current Hobart College. LeClair maintains the Blackwell Web Site at Hobart and William Smith Colleges. She has also written magazine articles on Blackwell and assists students and community members who are researching Blackwell's life.

Justin White has been a lifelong resident of Oswego, NY. He is a graduate of St. Bonaventure University in Allegany, NY. For many years he has studied the life of Oswego native Dr. Mary E. Walker, and given several presentations on her life. For nine years he worked on the staff of the Oswego County Historical Society. He currently works in the Oswego County Archives and has served as the appointed historian for the town of Oswego since 2001. As president of the Heritage Foundation of Oswego County, White is actively involved in the preservation and promotion of the historical, architectural and environmental resources of the Oswego area.

(Continued)

Susan Keeter MFA is a portrait painter and children's book illustrator, as well as a staff member at SUNY Upstate Medical University, home of the medical college where Dr. Sarah Loguen Fraser received her education. In 2000, the Syracuse Medical Alumni Association commissioned Keeter to paint the portrait of Dr. Loguen in honor of the 150th anniversary of her birth. In preparation, Keeter did research which led her to find a distant descendant and to study many special collections including those at Howard University. She has written on Dr. Sarah Loguen for *SUNY Upstate Medical University Outlook*. Keeter lives across the street from the site of Dr. Loguen's 1903 home and blocks from her childhood home. She gives inspiring talks on Dr. Loguen at schools and community groups and describes herself as profoundly honored to have the opportunity to celebrate the life of one of the nation's first African American women physicians.

INDEX

BLACKWELL ESSAY (pp.1-42)

WALKER ESSAY (pp.43-86)

LOGUEN FRASER ESSAY
(pp. 87-130)

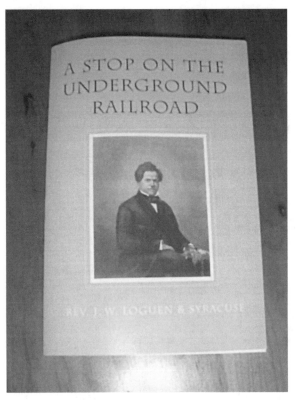